ECHO
MADE EASY

D1394129

First published in the UK by

Anshan Ltd
in 2005
6 Newlands Road
Tunbridge Wells
Kent TN4 9AT, UK

Tel/Fax: +44 (0)1892 557767
E-mail: info@anshan.co.uk
www.anshan.co.uk

ISBN 1 904798 276

British Library Cataloguing in Publication Data
A catalogue record for this book is available from the British Library

Printed in India by Gopsons Papers Ltd., A-14, Sector 60,Noida

*To
My Father
Mr PP Luthra
who made me
&
to
My Mother
Ms Prem Luthra
whose fond memories
always guide me*

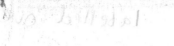

PREFACE

Ultrasound has revolutionized clinical practice by providing the fifth dimension to physical examination after inspection, palpation, percussion and auscultation. Echocardiography is the application of ultrasound for examining the heart. It is a practically useful, widely available, cost-effective and non-invasive diagnostic tool. Usage of echo is rapidly expanding with more and more clinicians requesting for and interpreting it to solve vexing clinical dilemmas.

While I was preparing the manuscript of this book, many a time two questions crossed my mind. First, Is such a book really required? And second, —Am I the right person to write it? At the end of the day, I somehow managed to convince myself that a precise and practical account of echocardiography is indeed required and that an academic physician like myself can do justice to this highly technical subject.

The book begins with the basic principles of ultrasound and Doppler and the clinical applications of various echo-modalities including 2-D echo, M-mode scan, Doppler echo and colour-flow mapping. This is followed by an account of different echo-windows and normal echo-views along with normal values and dimensions. The echo features of various forms of heart disease such as congenital, valvular, coronary and hypertensive disorders are individually discussed. Due emphasis has been laid on pitfalls in diagnosis, differentiation between seemingly similar findings, their causation and their clinical relevance. Understandably, figures and diagrams can never create the impact of dynamic echo display on the video-screen. Nevertheless, they have been specially created to leave a long-lasting visual impression on the mind. In keeping with the spirit of simplicity, difficult topics like complex congenital cardiac disease, prosthetic heart valves and transoesophageal echocardiography have been purposely excluded.

This book is particularly meant for students of cardiology as well as keen established clinicians wanting to know more about echo. If I can coax some physicians like myself to integrate echocardiography into their day-to-day clinical practice, I will feel genuinely elated for a mission successfully accomplished.

Atul Luthra

ACKNOWLEDGEMENTS

I am extremely grateful to:
- My school teachers who helped me to acquire command over spoken and written English language.
- My professors at medical college who taught me the science and art of clinical medicine.
- My heart patients whose echocardiograms stimulated my grey matter and made me wiser.
- Authors of textbooks on echocardiography which I referred to liberally while writing this book.
- M/s Jaypee Brothers Medical Publishers (P) Ltd who felt confident to assign this project to me and provided expert editorial assistance at all stages.
- My wife Arti and daughters Ankita and Aastha who left me to myself while I was preparing and proof-reading the manuscript.

CONTENTS

Contents

CHAPTER ONE

WHAT IS AN ECHO?

PRINCIPLE OF ULTRASOUND

- Sound is a mechanical disturbance transmitted through a medium which may be gas, liquid or solid. Every sound has a frequency, a velocity and an intensity.

- Frequency of sound is the number of times per second, sound undergoes a cycle of rise and fall. It is expressed in cycles per second, or Hertz (Hz) and multiples thereof. 1Hz is 1 cycle per second and units of frequency are kilo Hz (kHz -10^3 Hz) and mega Hz (MHz -10^6 Hz). Frequency is appreciated as the pitch of sound by the listener.

- Wavelength is the distance travelled by sound in one cycle. Frequency and wavelength are interrelated. Since sound travels a fixed distance in one second, more the cycles in a second (greater the frequency), shorter is the wavelength. Therefore, Velocity = Frequency × Wavelength (Fig. 1.1).

- Velocity of sound is expressed in meters per second or m/sec and is determined by the nature of the medium through which sound propagates. In soft tissue, the speed of sound is 1540 m/sec.

- Intensity of sound is nothing but its loudness or audibility expressed in decibels. Higher the intensity of sound, greater is the distance up to which it is audible.

- Sound of a frequency greater than what can be perceived by the human ear (more than 20 kHz) is called ultrasound. The technique of using ultrasound to examine the heart is known as echocardiography or ECHO.

- Ultrasound relies on the property of certain crystals to transform electrical current of varying voltage into

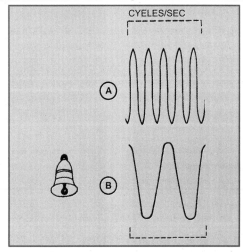

Fig. 1.1: Relationship between frequency and wave-length:
A. Higher frequency, shorter wave-length,
B. Lower frequency, longer wave-length

mechanical oscillations or ultrasound waves. This is known as the piezoelectric effect (Fig. 1.2). When electrical current is passed through a piezoelectric crystal, the crystal vibrates. This generates ultrasound waves which are transmitted through the body by the transducer which houses several such crystals. Most of these ultrasound waves are scattered or absorbed by tissues while a small proportion is reflected back to the transducer. Reflected ultrasound again distorts the piezoelectric crystals and produces an electrical current. The reflected signal gives information about the depth and nature of the tissue studied. Most of the reflection occurs at interfaces between tissues

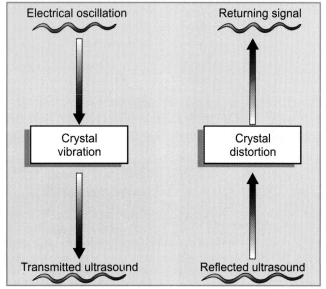

Fig. 1.2: The piezoelectric effect in ultrasound

having different density and thus different echo-reflectivity.

- The magnitude of the electrical current produced by the reflected ultrasound determines the intensity and echodensity on the display screen. On the grey-scale, high reflectivity (e.g. from bone) is white low reflectivity (e.g. from muscle) is grey, and no reflection (e.g. from air) is black.

- The location of the image produced by the reflected ultrasound depends upon the time lag between transmission and reflection of ultrasound. Deeper structures are shown on the lower portion of the display screen while superficial structures are shown

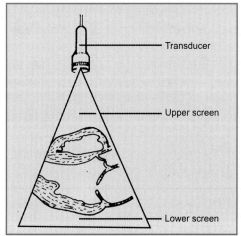

Fig. 1.3: The transducer is at the apex of image:
A. Right ventricle in upper part of screen,
B. Left ventricle in lower part of screen

on the upper portion of the screen. This is because the transducer position is always at the apex of the image (Fig. 1.3).

- When ultrasound is transmitted through a uniform medium, it maintains its original direction and get progressively scattered and absorbed. When ultrasound waves generated by the transducer encounter an interface between tissues of different density and thus different echo-reflectivity, some of the ultrasound waves are reflected back. It is these reflected ultrasound waves that are collected by the transducer and analysed by the echo-machine.

- The wavelength of sound is the ratio between velocity and frequency (Wavelength = Velocity/Frequency). Since wavelength and frequency are inversely

Table 1.1: Features and applications of ultrasound probes having different frequency				
Frequency (MHz)	Penetration	Resolution	Study depth	Age group
2.5-3.5	good	less	deep	adults
5.0-7.5	less	good	superficial	children

related, higher the frequency of ultrasound, shorter is the wavelength. Shorter the wavelength, higher is the image resolution and lesser is the penetration. Therefore, high frequency probes (5.0 to 7.5 MHz) provide better resolution when applied for superficial structures and in children (see Table 1.1). Conversely lower the frequency of ultrasound, longer is the wavelength. Longer the wavelength, lower is the image resolution and greater is the tissue penetration. Therefore, low frequency probes (2.5 to 3.5 MHz) provide better penetration when applied for deeper structures and in adults (see Table 1.1).

PRINCIPLE OF DOPPLER

- The Doppler effect is present and used by us in everyday life, even if we don't realise it. Imagine an automobile sounding the horn and moving towards you, going past you and then away from you. The pitch of the horn sound is higher when it approaches you (higher frequency) than when it goes away from you (lower frequency). The change of frequency (Doppler shift) depends upon the speed of the automobile and the original frequency of the horn sound.

- Ultrasound reflected back from a tissue interface gives information about the depth and echo-reflectivity of the tissue being studied. On the other hand, Doppler utilizes ultrasound reflected back by moving red blood cells (RBCs). The Doppler principle is used to derive the velocity of blood flow. Flow velocity is derived from the change of frequency that occurs between transmitted (original) and reflected (observed) ultrasound. The shift of frequency (Doppler shift) is proportional to ratio of velocity of blood to speed of sound and to the original frequency. It is calculated from the following formula:

$$F_D = \frac{V}{C} \times F_o$$

F_D is Doppler shift

F_o is original frequency
V is velocity of blood
C is speed of sound

Therefore,

$$V = \frac{F_D \times C}{F_o}$$

A further refinement of this formula is:

$$V = \frac{F_D \times C}{2 F_o \times Cos\theta}$$

- The original frequency (F_o) is multiplied by 2 since Doppler shift occurs twice during forward transmission as well as during backward reflection. Cosine thita ($Cos\theta$) is applied as a correction for the angle between the ultrasound beam and blood flow. $Cos\theta$ = 1 if beam is parallel to direction of blood flow and maximum velocity is observed. $\cos\theta = 0$ if beam is perpendicular to direction of blood flow and zero velocity is observed.

- It is noteworthy that for Doppler echo, maximum velocity information is obtained with the ultrasound beam aligned parallel to the direction of blood flow being studied. Otherwise, the peak velocity and consequently the pressure gradient (see below) are likely to be underestimated. This is in sharp contrast to conventional echo, where best image quality is obtained with the ultrasound beam aligned perpendicular to the structure being studied.

- Since the original frequency value ($2\ F_o$) is in the denominator of the velocity equation, it is important to remember that maximum velocity information is obtained using a low frequency generating transducer (around 2 MHz).

- There is a direct relationship between the peak flow velocity through a stenotic valve and the pressure gradient across it. Understandably, when the valve orifice is small, blood flow has to accelerate in order to eject the same stroke volume. This increase in velocity can be measured using Doppler echo. The pressure gradient across the valve can be calculated using the simplified Bernaulli equation:

$$\Delta P = 4\ V^2$$

when P is pressure gradient (in mm Hg)

V is peak flow velocity (in m/sec)

- This equation is frequently used during Doppler evaluation of stenotic valves, regurgitant lesions and intracardiac shunts. The velocity information provided by Doppler echo complements the anatomical information provided by M-mode and 2-D echocardio-graphy.

- Analysis of the returning Doppler signal not only provides information about flow velocity but also about flow direction. By convention, velocities towards the transducer are displayed above the baseline (positive deflection) and velocities away from the transducer are displayed below the baseline (negative deflection) (Fig. 1.4).

- The returning Doppler signal is a spectral trace of velocity display on a time axis. The area under curve (AUC) of the spectral trace is known as the flow velocity integral (FVI) of that velocity display. The value of FVI is determined by peak flow velocity and ejection time. It can be calculated by the computer of most echo machines.

- Careful analysis of the spectral trace of velocity also gives densitometric information. Density relates to the number of RBCs moving at a given velocity. When

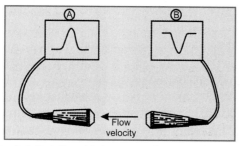

Fig. 1.4: Relationship between direction of flow and polarity of deflection:
A. Towards the transducer, positive deflection,
B. Away from the transducer, negative deflection

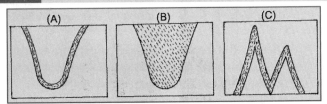

Fig. 1.5: Various patterns of blood flow on Doppler:
A. Laminar flow across normal aortic valve,
B. Turbulent flow across stenotic aortic valve,
C. Normal flow pattern across mitral valve

blood flow is smooth or laminar, most RBCs are travelling at the same velocity, accelerating and decelerating simultaneously. The spectral trace then has a thin outline form with very few RBCs travelling at other velocities (Figs 1.5A and C). This is known as low variance of velocities. When blood flow is turbulent as across stenotic valves, there is a wide distribution of RBCs velocities and the Doppler signal appears "filled in" (Fig. 1.5B). This is known as high variance of velocities, "spectral broadening" or increased "band width". It is to be borne in mind that turbulence and spectral broadening are often associated with but not synonymous with a high velocity signal.

- The intensity of the Doppler signal is represented on the grey-scale as increasing shades of grey. Maximum number of RBCs travelling at a particular velocity cast a dark shade on the spectral trace. Few RBCs travelling at a higher velocity cast a lighter shade. This is seen best on the Doppler signal from a stenotic valve. The spectral display is most dense near the baseline reflecting most RBCs moving above and below the valve at a low velocity. Few RBCs

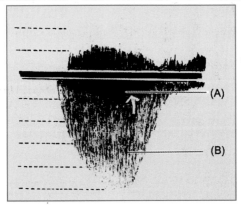

Fig. 1.6: Continuous wave Doppler signal from a stenotic valve showing turbulent flow: A. Most RBCs moving at low velocity, B. Few RBCs moving at high velocity

accelerating through the stenotic valve are at a high velocity (Fig. 1.6).

- The Doppler echo modes used clinically are continuous wave (CW) Doppler and pulsed wave (PW) Doppler. In CW Doppler, two piezoelectric crystals are used, one transmitting continuously and the other receiving continuously without any time delay. It can measure high velocities but it cannot precisely localize a signal which may originate from anywhere along the length or width of the ultrasound beam.

- In PW Doppler, a single piezoelectric crystal is used to transmit ultrasound and then to receive it after a preset time delay. PW Doppler can precisely localize the site of origin of a velocity signal. For this, a 'sample volume' is placed over the 2-D image at the region of interest. The 'sample volume' can be moved up and

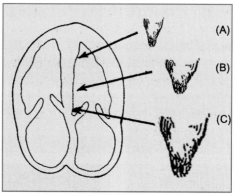

Fig. 1.7: Pulsed wave Doppler signal from various levels in the left ventricle: A. LV apex, B. Mid LV, C. Sub-aortic

down from one region to the other until a maximum velocity signal is obtained (Fig. 1.7). Because of the time delay in receiving the reflected ultrasound signal, PW Doppler cannot accurately detect high velocities exceeding 2 m/sec. However, PW Doppler provides a better quality of spectral tracings than does CW Doppler (Fig. 1.8).

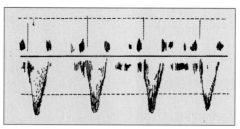

Fig. 1.8: Pulsed wave Doppler signal from a regurgitant valve showing laminar flow

- In the PW Doppler mode, the pulse repetition frequency (PRF) should be greater than twice the frequency of ultrasound being measured. This is known as the Nyquist Limit. If the PRF is less than this, the phenomenon of aliasing occurs. Aliasing is an artificial reversal of velocity and distortion of the reflected signal. Aliasing can be overcome by one of the following methods:
  - using a lower frequency probe.
  - reducing the depth of interrogation
  - shifting the baseline of spectral display

CHAPTER TWO

THE MODALITIES OF ECHO

The following modalities of echo are used clinically:

I. Conventional echo
   A. Two-dimensional echo (2-D echo)
   B. Motion-mode echo (M-mode echo)
II. Doppler echo
   A. Continuous wave (CW) Doppler
   B. Pulsed wave (PW) Doppler
   C. Colour flow (CF) Mapping

Different echo modalities are not mutually exclusive but complement each other and are often used together. All of them follow the same principle of ultrasound but differ with respect to the manner in which reflected sound waves are collected and analysed.

CONVENTIONAL ECHO

Two-Dimensional Echo (2-D Echo)

- Ultrasound reflected from a tissue interface distorts the piezoelectric crystal and generates an electric signal. The electric signal produces a dot (spot) on the display screen. The density and position of the dot (spot) is determined by nature and depth of the tissue studied.
- To create a 2-D image, the ultrasound beam has to be swept across the area of interest. Ultrasound is transmitted along several (about 90-120) scan lines over a wide (about 90°) arc and many (about 20-30) times per second. The combination of reflected ultrasound signals builds up an image on the display screen. Production of images in quick succession creates a 'real-time' image of moving structures. Any

image frame can be frozen, studied on the screen or printed out on thermal paper or X-ray film.

- 2-D echo is useful to evaluate the anatomy of the heart and the relationship between different structures. Intracardiac masses and extracardiac pericardial abnormalities can be noted. The motion of the walls of ventricles and cusps of valves is visualized (Fig. 2.1). Thickness of ventricular walls and dimensions of chambers can be measured and stroke volume, ejection fraction and cardiac output can be calculated. 2-D image is also used to place the 'cursor line' for M-mode echo and to position the 'sample volume' for Doppler echo.

Motion-Mode Echo (M-mode Echo)

- To create a M-mode image, ultrasound is transmitted and received along only one scan line. This is obtained by applying a cursor line to the 2-D image and aligning it perpendicularly to the structure being studied. For this, the transducer is angulated till the cursor line is perpendicular to the image.
- Since only one scan line is imaged, M-mode echo provides substantially greater sensitivity than 2-D echo for recording moving structures. It produces a graph of depth and strength of reflection against time. Motion and thickness of ventricular walls, changing size of cardiac chambers and opening and closure of valves is better displayed (Fig. 2.2). Simultaneous ECG recording facilitates accurate timing of cardiac events. Similarly, the flow pattern on colour flow mapping can be timed in relation to the cardiac cycle.

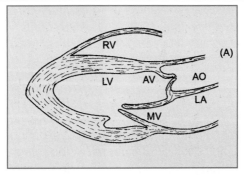

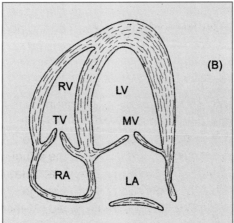

Fig. 2.1: Two-dimensional echo (2-D echo):
A. Parasternal long-axis (PLAX) view,
B. Apical 4-chamber (AP4CH) view

DOPPLER ECHO

Continuous Wave (CW) Doppler

- CW Doppler transmits and receives ultrasound continuously. It can measure high velocities without

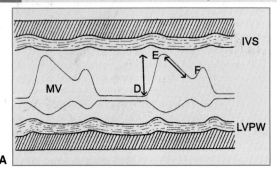

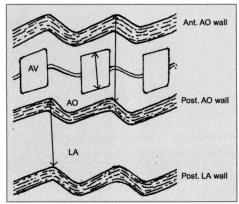

Fig. 2.2: Motion-mode echo (M-mode echo):
A. Mitral valve (MV) level,
B. Aortic valve (AV) level

any upper limit and is not hindered by the phenomenon of aliasing. However, CW Doppler cannot
precisely localize a signal which may originate
anywhere along the length or width of the ultrasound
beam (Fig. 2.3).

- This Doppler modality is used for rapid scanning of
  the heart in search of high velocity signals and

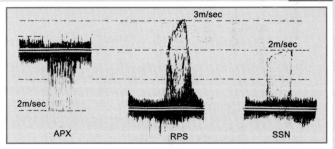

Fig. 2.3: Continuous wave (CW) Doppler signal from a stenosed aortic valve. Maximum velocity 3 m/sec

abnormal flow patterns. Since the Doppler frequency shift is in the audible range, the audio signal is used to angulate and rotate the transducer in order to obtain the best visual display. CW Doppler display forms the basis for placement of "sample volume" to obtain PW Doppler spectral tracing.

- CW Doppler is used for grading the severity of valvular stenosis and assessing the degree of valvular regurgitation. Intracardiac left-to-right shunt such as through a ventricular septal defect can be quantified. Using CW Doppler signal of tricuspid valve inflow, the pulmonary arterial pressure can be estimated.

Pulsed Wave (PW) Doppler

- PW Doppler transmits ultrasound in pulses and waits to receive the returning ultrasound after each pulse. Because of the time delay in receiving the reflected signal, which limits the rate of sampling, it cannot detect high velocities. At velocities exceeding 2 m/sec., there occurs a reversal of flow known as the

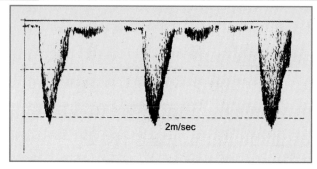

Fig. 2.4: Pulsed wave (PW) Doppler signal from a stenosed aortic valve. Maximum velocity 2 m/sec

phenomenon of aliasing. However, PW Doppler provides better quality spectral tracings than CW Doppler, which are more useful for calculations (Fig. 2.4).

• PW Doppler modality is used to localize velocity signals and abnormal flow patterns picked up by CW Doppler and colour flow mapping, respectively. The mitral valve inflow signal is used for the assessment of left ventricular diastolic dysfunction. The aortic valve outflow signal is used for the calculation of stroke volume and cardiac output.

Colour Flow (CF) Mapping

• Colour flow mapping is an automated 2-D version of PW Doppler. It calculates blood flow velocity and direction at multiple points along a scan line. A number of scan lines are used during CF mapping. The velocity and direction information is colour-encoded and superimposed on the 2-D image (Fig. 2.5).

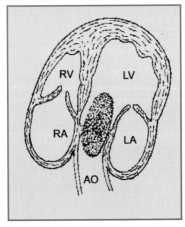

Fig. 2.5: Colour flow (CF) map of high velocity
signal across a stenosed aortic valve

By convention, velocities towards the transducer are
displayed in shades of red and those away in shades
of blue. This is known as the BART rule: Blue Away,
Red Towards.

- Higher velocities are shown in progressively lighter
colour shades, or as changes of hue. Low velocities
are dull and dark while high velocities are bright and
light. Above a threshold velocity, a reversal of colour
occurs which is the counterpart of aliasing on PW
Doppler. Areas of high turbulence or regions of flow
acceleration are depicted in green. An inadequate
echo window, malalignment of the transducer, a weak
flow signal and low gain setting are some of the
causes of a missed (false negative) colour flow map.

- This echo modality is used to screen for high velocity
signals and abnormal flow patterns from regurgitant

valves and left-to-right shunts. Areas of turbulence can be precisely localized and the Doppler beam can be aligned accordingly. Colour flow mapping also provides quantitative information. The area of a colour flow jet corresponds to the degree of valvular regurgitation and the width of the jet across a shunt approximates the size of the septal defect.

CLINICAL APPLICATIONS

2-D Echo

- anatomy of heart and structural relationships
- intracardiac masses and pericardial abnormalities
- motion of ventricular walls and valvular leaflets
- wall thickness, chamber volume and ejection fraction
- calculation of stroke volume and cardiac output
- architecture of valve leaflets and size of orifice
- positioning for M-mode and Doppler echo

M-mode Echo

- cavity size, wall thickness and muscle mass.
- excursion of ventricular walls and valvular cusps.
- timing of cardiac events with simultaneous ECG
- timing of flow pattern with colour flow mapping

CW Doppler

- grading the severity of valvular stenosis
- assessing degree of valvular regurgitation
- quantifying the pulmonary artery pressure
- scanning the heart for high velocity signal

PW Doppler

- assessment of left ventricular diastolic dysfunction
- calculation of stroke volume and cardiac output
- estimation of orifice area of stenotic aortic valve
- localization of flow pattern seen on CF mapping
- localization of signal picked up on CW Doppler
- obtaining good quality spectral tracing for calculations

CF Mapping

- screening for abnormal flow in valve regurgitation or left-to-right shunt
- quantitative assessment of abnormal flow pattern by jet area and width.

CHAPTER THREE

THE ECHO WINDOWS

TRANSTHORACIC ECHO

- Conventional echocardiography is performed from the anterior chest wall (precordium) and is known as transthoracic echo. Echocardiography can also be performed from the oesophagus which is known as transoesophageal echo.

- For transthoracic echo, the subject is asked to lie in the semirecumbent position on his or her left side with the head elevated. The left arm is tucked under the head and the right arm lies along the right side of the body. This position enlarges the 'windows' through which echocardiography can be performed while most of the heart is masked from the ultrasound beam by ribs and lungs. Better images are obtained during expiration when there is least 'air-tissue' interface.

- Ultrasound is transmitted from a transducer or probe having a frequency of 2.5 to 3.5 MHz for echo in adults. This frequency is used to study deep seated structures because of better penetration. A transducer frequency of 5.0 MHz is suitable for paediatric echo since the heart is more superficial in children. Ultrasound jelly is applied on the transducer and it is placed on the chest at the site of an "echo window". Most of the time, the left parasternal and apical windows are routinely used. The transducer has a line or dot to help orient it into the correct position for obtaining different echo views. The transducer is variably positioned for different echo images, angulated to bring into focus the structure of interest and rotated to fine-tune the image.

- Standard positions on the chest wall are used for placement of the transducer which are called "echo windows" (Fig. 3.1). These are:
  1. Left parasternal
  2. Apical
  3. Sub-costal
  4. Right parasternal
  5. Suprasternal

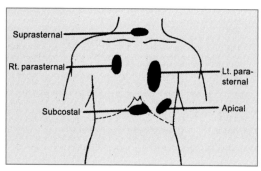

Fig. 3.1: The various echo "windows"

- Standard transducer positions are important for two main reasons:
  1. Penetration by ultrasound is good without much masking of image or absorption of ultrasound by ribs and lungs.
  2. Standardized echo images can be compared with studies performed by different observers or on different occasions.
- Transthoracic echo may be technically difficult to perform in the following situations:
  1. Severe morbid obesity

2. Chest wall deformity
3. Emphysema or lung fibrosis

Parasternal Long-Axis View (PLAX View) (Fig. 3.2)

Transducer position: left sternal edge ; 2nd - 4th i-c space
Marker dot direction: points towards right shoulder.

Structures seen:
ascending aorta
aortic valve
left atrium
mitral valve
left ventricle
IV septum
LV posterior wall
right ventricle
Most echo studies
begin with this view.

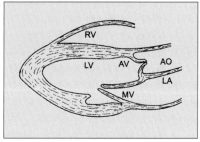

Fig. 3.2: The parasternal long-axis (PLAX) view

It sets the stage for subsequent echo views.

Parasternal Short-Axis Views (PSAX Views) (Fig. 3.3)

Transducer position:
left sternal edge ; 2nd – 4th i-c space
Marker dot direction:
points towards left shoulder
(90° clockwise from PLAX view)
By tilting the transducer on an axis between the left
hip and right shoulder, short-axis views are obtained at
different levels, from the aorta to the LV apex. This
angulation of the transducer from the base to apex of

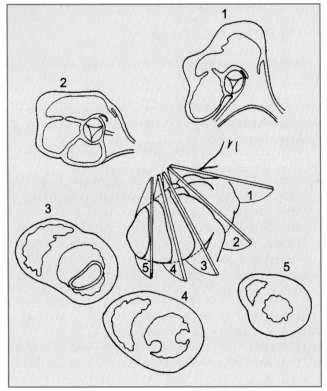

Fig. 3.3: The parasternal short-axis (PSAX) views

the heart for short-axis views is known as "bread-loafing". Short axis sections are taken at the following levels:

 pulmonary artery level
 aortic valve level
 mitral valve level
 papillary muscle level
 ventricular level

Pulmonary Artery (PA) Level (Fig. 3.4)

Structures seen: pulmonary artery
      pulmonary valve
      RV outflow tract

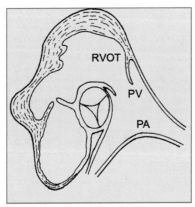

Fig. 3.4: PSAX view: pulmonary artery (PA) level

Aortic Valve (AV) Level (Fig. 3.5)

Structure seen:
  aortic valve cusps
  left atrium
  interatrial septum
  tricuspid valve
  RV outflow tract

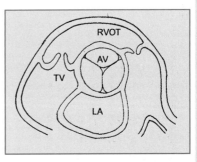

Fig. 3.5: PSAX view: aortic valve
(AV) level

Mitral Valve (MV) Level (Fig. 3.6)

Structures seen:
mitral valve orifice
mitral valve leaflets
interventricular septum

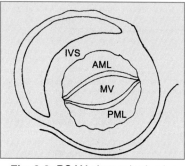

Fig. 3.6: PSAX view: mitral valve
(MV) level

Papillary Muscle (PM) Level (Fig. 3.7)

Structures seen:
anterolateral PM
(3 o'clock)
posteromedial PM
(7 o'clock)
LV wall thickness
regional wall motion.

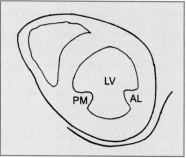

Fig. 3.7: PSAX view: papillary
muscle (PM) level

For apical views, the subject turns back rightwards from the left lateral position and lies supine.

Apical 4-Chamber View (AP4CH View) (Fig. 3.8)

Transducer position: apex of the heart
Marker dot direction: points towards left shoulder

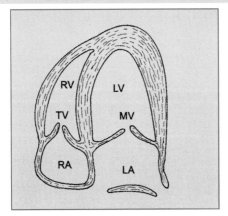

Fig. 3.8: Apical 4-chamber (AP4CH) view

Structures seen: right and left ventricle
right and left atrium
mitral and tricuspid valves
IA septum and IV septum
left ventricular apex
LV lateral wall

Apical 5-Chamber View (AP5CH view) (Fig. 3.9)

Transducer position: same as AP4CH view
Marker dot direction: same as AP4CH view

The AP5CH view is obtained from the AP4CH view by slight anterior angulation of the transducer towards the chest wall. The 5th chamber added is the left ventricular outflow tract (LVOT)

Structures seen: Same as AP4CH view +
aortic valve and
ascending aorta.

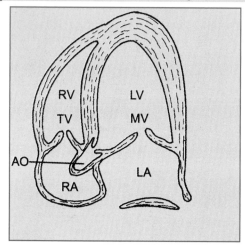

Fig. 3.9: Apical 5-chamber (AP5CH) view

Apical 2-Chamber View (AP2CH View) (Fig. 3.10) or Apical Long-Axis View

Transducer position: apex of the heart
Marker dot direction: points towards left side of neck
(45° anticlockwise from AP4CH view)
Structures seen: LV anterior wall
                   LV inferior wall

Sub-Costal 4-Chamber View (SC4CH View)

For subcostal view, the position of the subject is different
from that used to obtain parasternal and apical views.
The subject lies supine with the head held slightly low
(no pillow). With the feet on the bed, the knees are

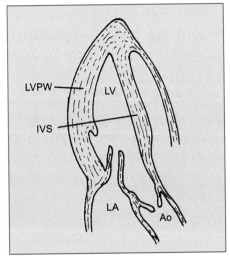

Fig. 3.10: Apical long-axis (APLAX) view

slightly elevated (with pillow). Better images are obtained with the abdomen relaxed and during inspiration.

Transducer position: under the xiphisternum

Marker dot position: points towards left shoulder

Structures seen: same as in AP4CH view.

The subcostal view is particularly useful when transthoracic echo is technically difficult because of severe obesity, chest wall deformity, emphysema or pulmonary fibrosis.

The following structures are better seen from the subcostal view than from the apical 4-chamber view:

inferior vena cava and hepatic veins

descending abdominal aorta

interatrial septum

pericardial effusion

Suprasternal View

For suprasternal view, the subject lies supine with the neck hyperextended by placing a pillow under the shoulders. The head is rotated slightly towards the left. The position of arms or legs and the phase of respiration have no bearing on this echo window.

Transducer position: suprasternal notch
Marker dot direction: points towards left jaw
Structure seen: arch of aorta.

Right Parasternal View

For right parasternal view, the subject lies in the semi-recumbent position on his or her right side. The right arm is tucked under the head and the left arm lies along the left side of the body. In other words, this position is the mirror-image of that used for the left parasternal view.

Transducer position: right sternal edge; 2nd-4th i-c space
Marker dot direction: points towards left shoulder
Structures seen: aortic valve and ascending aorta

TRANSOESOPHAGEAL ECHO

Principle

During echocardiography, a balance has to be struck between tissue penetration and image resolution. Low frequency transducers used for transthoracic echo have good penetration (less attenuation) but relatively poor resolution. On the other hand, high frequency transducers have poor penetration (more attenuation) but better resolution.

Anatomically speaking, the oesophagus in its mid-course is strategically located posterior to the heart and anterior to the descending aorta. This provides an opportunity to examine the heart and related structures with a high frequency transducer positioned in the oesophagus for better image resolution. The technique is known as transoesophageal echo.

Technique

The transducer is mounted onto a scope similar to that employed for upper gastrointestinal endoscopy and advanced to various depths in the oesophagus. By manoeuvring the transducer and the angle of ultrasound beam from controls on the handle, different views of the heart are obtained. This 'back-door' approach to echocardiography has both advantages and dis-advantages.

Advantages

1. Useful alternative to transthoracic echo if the latter is technically difficult due to obesity, chest wall deformity, emphysema or pulmonary fibrosis.
2. Useful complement to transthoracic echo because of better image quality and resolution. This is because of two reasons:
   a. Lack of interference between the ultrasound beam and ribs
   b. Greater proximity to the heart and therefore the ability to use higher frequency probe with better image resolution.

3. Useful supplement to transthoracic echo which cannot examine the posterior aspect of the heart for left atrial appendage, descending aorta and pulmonary veins.

Disadvantages

1. It is an invasive procedure which is uncomfortable to the patient, more time consuming and carries a small risk of complications such as oesophageal trauma, arrhythmias and laryngo-bronchospasm.
2. It requires short-term sedation, oxygen administration and ECG monitoring since there are chances of hypoxia, arrhythmia and angina. Rarely, respiratory depression or allergic reaction may occur due to the sedative.
3. It is contraindicated in presence of dysphagia, oesaphageal varices, unstable cervical arthritis and severe pulmonary disease.

The transoesophageal echo (TOE) views are significantly different from standard transthoracic echo views and have to be learnt separately. It would be beyond the scope and against the philosophy of this book to understand and learn these views in detail. Nevertheless the indications for TOE are duly mentioned at appropriate places as, we go through the chapters of the book.

FUTURE DIRECTIONS IN ECHO

Myocardial Contrast Imaging

Techniques are being developed to improve assessment of myocardial perfusion, viability and function by use of sonicated radiographic contrast materials. Coronary flow can then be estimated by time-intensity curves of sonodensity.

Tissue Characterization

In this method, different radiofrequency values are assigned to tissues that are ischemic, viable and non-functional. Analysis of reflected frequencies can differentiate acute from chronic ischemia. Better visualization of the endocardial surface will improve assessment of dynamic function and wall motion.

3-D Echo Technology

Using computer software, 3-D representation of the left ventricle structure and function can be assessed. This avoids certain geometrical assumptions about the LV shape particularly if it has been distorted by prior infarction. Serial LV volumetric measurements in valvular regurgitation (MR, AR) can help proper timing of corrective surgery.

CHAPTER FOUR

NORMAL VIEWS AND VALUES

NORMAL ECHO

- The echocardiogram provides a substantial amount of structural and functional information about the heart. While still frames provide anatomical detail, dynamic images tell us about physiological function.
- Echocardiography is quite easy to understand since many echo features are based upon simple physical facts and physiological principles. Nevertheless, the value of information derived from echo depends heavily upon who has performed it. The quality of an echo is highly operator dependent and proportional to experience and skill.
- The abnormal can only be viewed in the light of the normal. Therefore, it is important to appreciate normal echo images and to be familiar with normal value ranges of dimensions and excursions.

SEQUENCE OF SCANNING

A suggested schematic for a systematic and detailed echocardiography study is as follows:
- Start with the parasternal long-axis view
- Make M-mode recording at 3 levels
  a. level of aortic valve
  b. level of mitral valve
  c. level of left ventricle
- Rotate the transducer by 90° clockwise. Angulate it from the base to apex to obtain short-axis views at 4 levels
  a. pulmonary artery level
  b. aortic valve level
  c. mitral valve level
  d. papillary muscle level

- Go on to the apical 4-chamber view. Measure ventricular volumes in systole diastole (to assess LV systolic function)
- Turn on the colour flow mapping for abnormal flow patterns due to valvular diseases or septal defects.
- Place the pulsed wave (PW) Doppler 'sample volume' in the LV cavity at the tips of MV leaflets in the diastolic position (to assess LV diastolic function)
- Angulate the transducer anteriorly to obtain the apical 5-chamber view. Place the 'sample volume' in the aortic valve to obtain the flow velocity integral (FVI). Calculate the stroke volume and thus the cardiac output.
- Use continuous wave (CW) Doppler to scan the apical 4-chamber view for high velocity signal, if abnormal flow pattern has been observed on colour flow mapping.
- Use pulsed wave (PW) Doppler to localize an abnormal flow pattern observed on colour flow mapping or a high velocity signal picked up on CW Doppler.
- Use other echo windows (subcostal, suprasternal and right parasternal) as and when indicated.
- Rotate the transducer by 45° anticlockwise and obtain the apical 2-chamber view.

WHAT IS NORMAL?

It must be borne in mind that normal value ranges of echo-derived dimensions, depend upon several factors. These factors include height, sex, age and physical training.

In general, normal values tend to be higher in the following subsets:

1. male gender
2. tall persons
3. trained athletes and
4. elderly individuals

Therefore, correction for these factors is made by indexing cardiac dimensions to body surface area (BSA) as follows:

$$BSA(m^2) = \sqrt{\frac{height(cm) \times weight(kg)}{3600}}$$

Normal dimensions are estimated from small populations of 'average' persons and may not apply to unusually small or tall subjects, to the elderly or to those of athletic built.

NORMAL VARIANTS

Some findings on echo may be normal and must be carefully understood to avoid overdiagnosis of a pathological cardiac condition in a normal subject (Fig. 4.1).

Normal Structures

- a moderator band may be seen in the apical one-third of the right ventricle, parallel to the plane of the tricuspid valve.
- a false tendon may be seen in the left ventricle, extending between the lateral papillary muscle and the IV septum.
- a Eustachian valve may be seen in the right atrium, guarding the opening of the inferiar vena cava into this chamber.

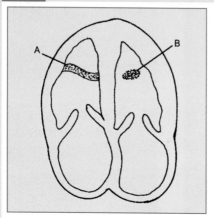

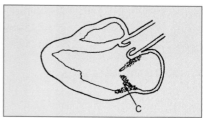

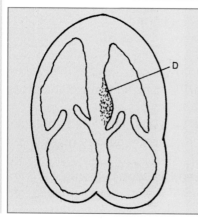

Fig. 4.1: Normal structural variants on echo:
A Moderator band in right ventricle.
B False tendon in the left ventricle,
C Mitral annular ring calcification,
D Sub-aortic bulging of IV septum

- a reverberation artefact may be seen in the left atrium, from a calcific mitral annulus or a prosthetic aortic valve.

Normal Flow Patterns

- Trivial tricuspid and pulmonary regurgitation are found in many subjects.
- Trivial mitral regurgitation is observed in some subjects
  Minor aortic regurgitation is more likely to be abnormal.

Normal Findings in Elderly

- Thickening of aortic valve leaflets without significant stenosis (misdiagnosed as aortic valve stenosis)
- Mitral annular ring calcification with some regurgitation (misdiagnosed as vegetation, thrombus or myxoma)
- Reduced LV compliance with A:E ratio > 1 on Doppler trace (misdiagnosed as left ventricular diastolic dysfunction)
- Localized subaortic bulging of the interventricular septum (misdiagnosed as asymmetric septal hypertrophy of HOCM).

NORMAL VALUES

- Most echo studies begin with the parasternal long-axis (PLAX) view. It sets the stage for subsequent echo views. Traditionally, dimensions are measured using M-mode scan (see below) which has better resolution than 2-D echo. However, despite this

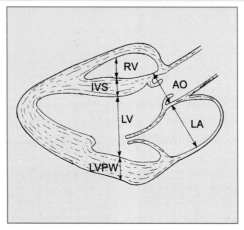

Fig. 4.2: Measurement of dimensions
from PLAX view

theoretical advantage, M-mode imaging may be inaccurate unless the cursor is placed perpendicular to the structure being measured. Practically speaking, this may not be always possible. In that case, measurements can instead be made from the 2-D image, PLAX view (Fig. 4.2).

- An experienced echocardiographer can often give a reasonably good visual assessment of LV systolic function from the PLAX view without actually taking measurements. However, this rough assessment may be unreliable for serial evaluation of LV function and when LV volumes critically influence the timing of a surgical intervention.
- The PLAX view gives a good visual impression of the motion of the interventricular septum (IVS) and the left ventricular posterior wall (LVPW) (Fig. 4.3).

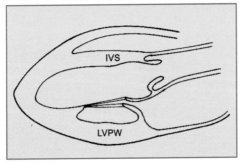

Fig. 4.3: Motion of IVS and LVPW seen on PLAX view

Several cardiac conditions can be readily diagnosed from the absolute and relative motion of these walls.

LVPW Motion

Reduced

LV posterior wall infarction
Dilated cardiomyopathy
Constrictive pericarditis

Exaggerated

with exaggerated IVS motion LV volume overload
with paradoxical IVS motion RV volume overload
with normal IVS motion MV paraprosthetic leak
with reduced IVS motion Septal wall infarction

IVS Motion

Reduced

Septal wall infarction
Hypertrophic myopathy
Dilated cardiomyopathy

Exaggerated

> LV volume overload
> Hyperdynamic state

Paradoxical

> RV volume overload
> Constrictive pericarditis
> Left bundle branch block
> After cardiac surgery

Parasternal Long-Axis View (PLAX View)

The PLAX view is used to measure the dimensions of the aortic annulus, sinus of Valsalva, aortic root and the anterior aortic swing (Fig. 4.4). Aortic valve orifice area can be calculated by the continuity equation.

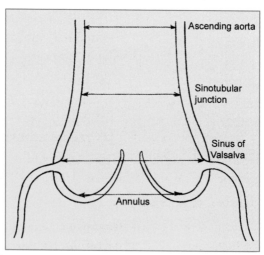

Fig. 4.4: Dimensions of proximal aorta from PLAX view

Normal aortic dimensions

Aortic annulus	17-25 mm
Sinus of Valsalva	22-36 mm
Sinotubular junction	18-26 mm
Aortic root (tubular)	20-37 mm
Anterior aortic swing	7-15 mm
Aortic valve orifice area	2.5-3.5 cm^2

M-mode Scan PLAX View

Aortic Valve Level (Fig. 4.5)

Aortic root diameter	20-37 mm
Aortic cusp separation	15-26 mm
Left atrial diameter	19-40 mm

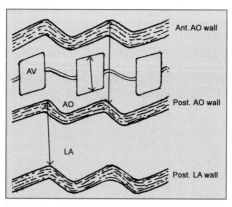

Fig. 4.5: M-mode scan from PLAX view—aortic valve level

Mitral Valve Level (Fig. 4.6)

AML D-E excursion	20-35 mm
AML E to F slope	18-120 mm/sec
E. point septal distance	less than 5 mm

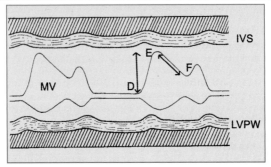

Fig. 4.6: M-mode scan from PLAX view—mitral valve level

Note: The diameter of the aortic root is measured between the leading edges of the anterior and posterior aortic walls. Similarly, the diameter of the left atrium is measured between the leading edges of the anterior and posterior atrial walls.

Ventricular Level (Fig. 4.7)

IV-septal thickness (diastolic)   6-12 mm
Posterior wall thickness (diastolic)   6-11 mm

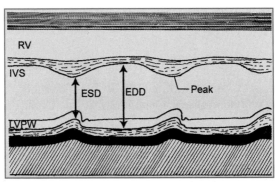

Fig. 4.7: M-mode scan from PLAX view—ventricular level

IV-septal excursion (systolic)	6-9 mm
Posterior wall excursion (systolic)	9-14 mm
LV dimension end-diastolic (LVEDD)	36-52 mm
end-systolic (LVESD)	24-42 mm

LV mass less than 134 g/m^2 (men)
         less than 110 g/m^2 (women)

RV internal dimension	7-23 mm
RV free-wall thickness	< 5 mm
LV fractional shortening	30-45%
LV ejection fraction	50-75%

Note: The dimensions of the left ventricle are measured at a level just below the free edge of the anterior mitral leaflet. This standardized level is important for serial comparative studies by the same or different observers on different occasions.

Parasternal Short-Axis View (PSAX View)

Pulmonary Artery Level

Pulmonary artery diameter = Aortic root diameter
Pulmonary valve outflow velocity 0.5-1.0 m/sec
                          (mean 0.75 m/sec)

Aortic Valve Level

Aortic root dimension	20-37 mm
Left atrial diameter	19-40 mm

Mitral Valve Level

Mitral valve orifice area 4-6 cm^2
(by planimetry method)

Papillary Muscle Level

LV A-P diameter   24-42 mm

Apical 4-Chamber View (AP4CH View)

LV volume
  end- diastolic (LVEDV) 85 ± 15 ml/m^2
  end- systolic (LVESV) 35 ± 5 ml/m^2
Mitral valve inflow velocity   0.6-1.4 m/sec
                               (mean 0.9 m/sec)
Tricuspid valve inflow velocity 0.3-0.7 m/sec
                               (mean 0.5 m/sec)

Apical 5-Chamber View (AP5CH View)

Aortic valve outflow velocity 0.9-1.8 m/sec
                               (mean 1.3 m/sec)
Stroke volume   32-48 ml/beat /m^2
Cardiac output   2.4-4.2 L/min/m^2

NORMAL VALVES

Mitral Valve

- The mitral valve consists of 2 leaflets namely, the anterior mitral leaflet (AML) and the posterior mitral leaflet (PML). Motion of both the leaflets is visualized by M-mode scanning from the PLAX view.
- The excursion of the AML can be divided into the following individual waves and slopes (Fig. 4.8):
  E wave   : anterior and posterior motion during diastole.
  D-E slope : anterior motion during rapid diastolic filling.

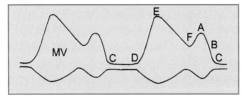

Fig. 4.8: M-mode tracing of mitral valve leaflets

E-F slope : posterior motion during end of diastolic period.

A wave   : anterior motion during atrial systolic contraction

B-C slope : posterior motion at onset of ventricular systole (isovolumic phase)

C-D slope : anterior motion during actual ventricular systole (ejection phase)

- The amplitude of motion of the PML is less than that of the AML and in a direction opposite to AML excursion.

Tricuspid Valve

- The tricuspid valve consists of 3 leaflets—a large anterior leaflet (ATL), a small septal leaflet (STL) and a tiny posterior leaflet (PTL). The ATL motion is visualized by M-mode scanning from the PLAX view in the right ventricle, anterior to the interventricular septum.
- The excursion of the ATL is very similar to that of the AML of mitral valve (see above) (Fig. 4.9).
- The STL is only recorded when there is either dilatation of the right ventricle or rotation of the heart due to emphysema and corpulmonale. The amplitude of motion of the STL is less than that of the ATL and in a direction opposite to ATL excursion.

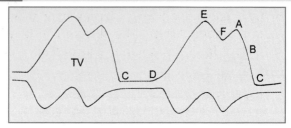

Fig. 4.9: M-mode tracing of tricuspid valve leaflets

* The PTL is not visualized on M-mode tracing of the valve.

Aortic Valve

* The aortic valve consists of 3 cusps—an anterior right coronary cusp (RCC), a posterior non-coronary cusp (NCC) and a middle left coronary cusp (LCC). The RCC and NCC are visualized by M-mode scanning from the PLAX view.
* During systole, the anterior and posterior cusps move away from each other towards the anterior and posterior aortic walls respectively. This creates a box-like systolic opening of the valve, in the shape of a parallelogram (Fig. 4.10).

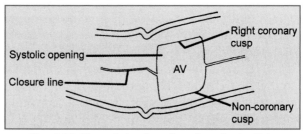

Fig. 4.10: M-mode tracing of aortic valve leaflets

- During diastole, the 3 cusps form a central closure line in the aortic lumen. The closure line is nearly equidistant from the anterior and posterior aortic walls.

Pulmonary Valve

- The pulmonary valve consists of 3 cusps—a posterior (left) cusp, an anterior cusp and a right cusp. The only cusp usually recordable by M-mode scanning from the PLAX view is the posterior (left) cusp. The anterior and right cusps are infrequently detected because of obliquity of the valve to ultrasound beam.
- The excursion of the posterior pulmonary leaflet can be divided into the following slopes (Fig. 4.11):

  a dip   : atrial contraction (presystole)

  B-C slope : systolic opening motion

  C-D slope : open valve during systole

  D-E slope : systolic closing motion

  E-F slope : diastolic posterior motion.

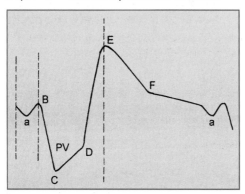

Fig. 4.11: M-mode tracing of pulmonary valve leaflet

CHAPTER FIVE

VENTRICULAR DYSFUNCTION

Assessment of ventricular function, particularly of the left ventricle, is one of the commonest and most important applications of echocardiography. Presence of left ventricular dysfunction is a reliable prognostic indicator in all forms of cardiac disease. It has important therapeutic implications and many a time, clinical management is altered when an abnormality is detected in ventricular function. Ventricular dysfunction can be classified into the following types:

1. Left ventricular systolic dysfunction
2. Left ventricular diastolic dysfunction
3. Right ventricular dysfunction

LV SYSTOLIC DYSFUNCTION

In order to understand LV systolic dysfunction, it is important to know the normal indices of ventricular function.

Normal Indices

LV wall thickness in diastole

6-12 mm Inter-Ventricular Septum (IVS)

6-11 mm LV Posterior Wall (LVPW)

LV wall excursion in systole

6-9 mm Inter-ventricular septum (IVS)

9-14 mm LV posterior wall (LVPW)

LV Internal dimension at end-systole

24-42 mm (LVESD)

at end-diastole

36-52 mm (LVEDD)

LV Internal volume at end-systole

35 ± 5 ml (LVESV)

at end - diastole
85 ± 15 ml (LVEDV)

Fractional shortening	30-45%
(% change in LV dimension)	
LV Ejection fraction	50-75%
(% change in LV volume)	

Echo Features of LV Systolic Dysfunction

M-Mode LV Level

- During ventricular systole, the interventricular septum (IVS) and the left ventricular posterior wall (LVPW) move towards each other. The amplitude of this motion is reduced in the presence of LV dysfunction (Fig. 5.1).

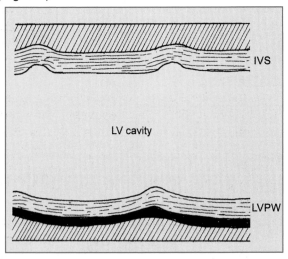

Fig. 5.1: M-mode scan from PLAX view at LV level showing: A. Reduced excursion of IV septum and LV posterior wall, B. Increased dimension of the left ventricular cavity

- LV internal dimension in end-systole (LVESD) and end-diastole (LVEDD) are measured on the M-mode tracing in the parasternal long-axis view (PLAX), at the level of mitral valve (MV) leaflet tips. Measurements are taken from the endocardial surface of the IVS to that of the LVPW. LV dimensions are increased in the presence of LV dysfunction.

- The percentage change in LV internal dimension between systole and diastole is called fractional shortening.

$$FS = \frac{LVEDD - LVESD}{LVEDD} \times 100\%$$

The normal range of fractional shortening is 30-45%. Reduced fractional shortening is an indicator of LV systolic dysfunction. However, in the presence of regional wall motion abnormality, the fractional shortening may not reliably reflect overall LV systolic performance.

- The normal volume of the left ventricle in end-diastole (LVEDV) is 85 ± 15 ml. A volume greater than 100 ml is indicative of LV systolic dysfunction either due to myocardial disease (cardiomyopathy/myocardial infarction) or volume overload of the ventricle (mitral /aortic regurgitation). The LV volume is derived from the 'cubed equation' $V = D^3$.

where V is the volume and D is the ventricular dimension measured by M-mode. This equation is based on the assumption that the LV cavity is ellipsoid in shape and the major axis is twice the minor axis (Fig. 5.2).

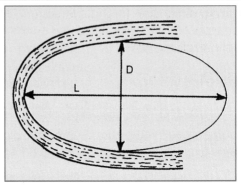

Fig. 5.2: Simulation of left ventricular cavity as ellipsoid. Major axis (L) is twice the minor axis (D). LV volume = D^3 from the cubed equation

- The percentage change in LV volume between systole and diastole is called ejection fraction

$$EF = \frac{LVEDV - LVESV}{LVEDV} \times 100\%$$

The normal range of ejection fraction is 50-75%. Reduced ejection fraction is an indicator of LV systolic dysfunction. However, the ejection fraction also depends upon ventricular loading conditions (preload and afterload).

- The normal thickness of the left ventricular walls, that is interventricular septum (IVS) and left ventricular posterior wall (LVPW) in diastole, is 6 to 12 mm. Walls thinner than 6 mm are due to stretching in cardiomyopathy or scarring due to prior myocardial infarction. Walls thicker than 12 mm indicate presence of ventricular hypertrophy. Normally, the walls should thicken in systole. Reduced systolic thickening of walls indicates presence of LV systolic dysfunction, either global (cardiomyopathy) or regional (myocardial infarction).

2-D Echo AP4CH View

2-D Echo can also be used to estimate LV volume in end-diastole (LVEDV) and end - systole (LVESV). This is done by tracing the LV endocardial borders of a systolic and a diastolic LV frame while the online computer software of the echo machine calculates the LV volume in systole and diastole. From these volumes, the ejection fraction can be calculated as mentioned above.

- The above method of calculating LV volume relies on manually tracing the ventricular endocardial outline. Alternatively, LV volume can be calculated totally by the computer using the Simpson's method. In this method the left ventricle is divided into 20 sections of known thickness. The computer takes multiple short-axis slices at different levels (Fig. 5.3). The volume of each slice is area multiplied by thickness.

Volume of each slice	$=$ Area $\times$ Thickness
Area of each slice	$= \pi (D/2)^2$
	D is diameter
Thickness of each slice	$= 1/20 \times$ LV length
LV volume	$=$ sum of volumes of all slices.

- The cardiac output can also be obtained using LV volumes by the following simple calculations:
  Stroke volume (SV) = LVEDV - LVESV
  Cardiac output = SV $\times$ Heart rate.

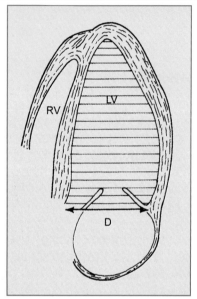

Fig. 5.3: Estimation of left ventricular volume by the Simpson's method. D is LV diameter at each level

Doppler Echo

- The cardiac output as an indicator of LV systolic function can be calculated from the peak aortic flow velocity (Vmax). This is obtained by Doppler display of aortic outflow from the apical 5 chamber (AP5CH) view (Fig. 5.4). Continuous wave (CW) Doppler is used to measure higher velocities and pulse wave (PW) Doppler for lower velocities. PW Doppler provides a better quality spectral velocity tracing.

  Before going into calculations of cardiac output, one must know the normal indices of ventricular ejection:

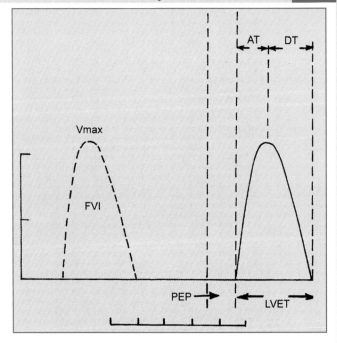

Fig. 5.4: Calculation of cardiac output from
peak aortic flow velocity (Vmax)
FVI = flow velocity integral
PEP = pre-ejection period
LVET = LV ejection time
AT   = acceleration time
DT   = deceleration time

Stroke volume = 32-48 ml / beat /m^2
Cardiac output = 2.8 - 4.2 L/ min /m^2
   (corrected for body surface area)
Doppler calculations.
Cardiac output = SV × HR

SV - stroke volume

HR - heart rate.

Stroke volume = CSA × FVI

CSA - cross-sectional area

FVI - flow velocity integral

$$CSA = \pi r^2 = \pi (D/2)^2 = \frac{22}{7} \times \frac{D^2}{4}$$

$$= 0.785 \, D^2$$

D = diameter of aortic annulus (Fig. 5.5)

$$FVI = \frac{PFV \times ET}{2 \rightarrow}$$

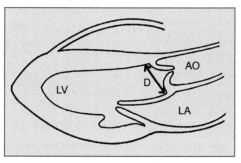

Fig. 5.5: Measuring diameter of aortic annulus (D) to calculate cross-sectional area (CSA) of the aortic valve

PFV— peak flow velocity (cm/sec)

ET—ejection time (sec/beat)

The FVI is calculated by the computer of most echo machines as the area under curve of aortic outflow velocity spectral display.

$$CO = 0.785 \, D^2 \times FVI \times HR$$

• Using similar calculations, the stroke volume of the right side of heart can be obtained using the peak pulmonary flow velocity (Vmax) and diameter of the pulmonary valve. Thereafter, the ratio of pulmonary flow (Q_p) to systemic flow (Q_s) which is the Q_p: Q_s ratio, can be calculated to quantify a cardiac shunt (see Congenital Heart Diseases)

Pitfalls in the Diagnosis of LV Systolic Dysfunction

- LV internal dimensions are taken between endocardial surfaces of IVS and LVPW. Errors in measurement may occur if a prominent papillary muscle or a calcified mitral annulus is mistaken for the endocardial surface of LVPW. As a differentiating feature, only the LVPW thickens in systole. Abnormal septal motion (e.g. LBBB) makes fractional shortening difficult to measure.
- The normal range for LVEDD and LVESD varies with a number of factors including age, sex, height and body habitus. This should always be borne in mind.
- Reduced LV systolic function is usually but not always associated with increased LV dimensions. For instance, a large akinetic segment of the LV wall following myocardial infarction may impair LV systolic function but LV dimensions may be within the normal range.
- An experienced echocardiographer can often give a reasonably good visual assessment of LV systolic function from the PLAX view, without actually taking measurements. However, this rough assessment may be unreliable for serial evaluation of LV function and when LV volumes critically influence the timing of a surgical intervention.

- There may be inter-observer and even more surprisingly, intra-observer variations in the measurement of LV dimensions, LV volumes and thus computing of fractional shortening and ejection fraction. Often these are due to variations in the frame frozen for calculations and in the delineation of the endocardial surface.

- While calculating LV volumes, certain geometrical assumptions are made about LV shape which are not always valid, particularly in a diseased heart. This often occurs in regional LV dysfunction. Post-infarction LV remodelling increases LV sphericity and causes alteration of the normal ellipse shape of the left ventricle.

- When assessing LV systolic function, one must allow for effects of volume loading and drug therapy. Fluid overload and antiarrhythmic drugs with negative ionotropy may further impair LV function.

- In presence of mitral regurgitation (MR), ejection fraction (EF) may be normal despite reduced contractility of the LV. This is because the left atrium offers less resistance to ejection than does the aorta. Conversely, in presence of aortic stenosis (AS), ejection fraction (EF) may be low despite normal contractility of the LV. This is because the left ventricle has to overcome a high transaortic resistance during ejection. Therefore, after surgery (valve repair or replacement) for MR, the EF falls and after surgery for AS, the EF rises.

- The calculation of cardiac output from peak aortic flow velocity by Doppler is invalid if the aortic valve is regurgitant or stenotic, because of an increased aortic flow velocity. The measurement of aortic valve diameter (D) at the aortic annulus is not only difficult but any inaccuracy is magnified since the D value is squared.

Causes of LV Systolic Dysfunction

Practically all forms of cardiac disease can ultimately culminate into LV systolic dysfunction. The prominent causes, in decreasing order of frequency are :
- Coronary artery disease
  — multiple infarcts, large infarct, triple vessel disease
- Hypertensive heart disease
  — decompensated stage of left ventricular hypertrophy.
- Valvular heart disease
  — mitral and aortic valve regurgitation with volume overload.
- Primary myocardial disease
  — dilated cardiomyopathy of varying etiology
- Congenital heart disease
  — left-to-right shunt due to a ventricular septal defect.

Clinical Significance of LV Systolic Dysfunction

- The presence of LV systolic dysfunction in any form of cardiac disease carries an adverse prognostic implication.
- Patients of coronary artery disease who have LV systolic dysfunction in addition to wall motion abnormalities have a lower survival rate and poorer

outcome after a revascularization procedure like by-pass surgery.

- When a patient of hypertension with left ventricular hypertrophy develops LV systolic dysfunction, it indicates the onset of decompensated stage of hypertensive heart disease.

- Volume overloading of the left ventricle due to valvular regurgitation or a left-to-right shunt will ultimately cause LV systolic dysfunction. Besides being a prognostic marker, onset of systolic dysfunction plays a crucial role in the timing of corrective surgery.

- Presence of LV systolic dysfunction is an important criteria for the diagnosis of dilated cardiomyopathy. Serial echocardiograms can not only assess the natural history of the disease but also the response to therapy.

- Subtle abnormalities of systolic function may not be obvious at rest but brought out by exertion or stress testing. Similarly, only minor systolic dysfunction may be observed after drug treatment of heart failure, which may have caused clinical improvement.

- Myocarditis is inflammation of the heart muscle often due to viral (Coxsackie B), bacterial (Mycoplasma) or parasitic (Lyme disease) infections. The echo features of myocarditis are similar to those of dilated cardiomyopathy with systolic and diastolic dysfunction and valvular regurgitation. Occasionally, regional wall motion abnormalities are noticed due to patchy inflammation. The differentiating features of myocarditis are a short history of febrile illness, ECG showing resting tachycardia with T wave inversion and serial echos showing rapidly changing LV function and degree of regurgitation.

LV DIASTOLIC DYSFUNCTION

In order to understand LV diastolic dysfunction, it is important to first understand the diastolic phase of the cardiac cycle. Diastole is divided into 4 discrete periods:

1. Isovolumic relaxation—AV closure to MV opening
2. Early rapid filling—from MV opening to end of filling
3. Diastasis phase—equilibration phase
4. Atrial systole—active atrial contraction

1 and 2 comprise the phase of myocardial relaxation which is an active energy dependent process.

3 and 4 comprise the phase of myocardial distensibility which is a passive stiffness dependant process

Therefore there are 2 patterns of diastolic dysfunction:

A. Slow-relaxation pattern
B. Restrictive pattern

Diastolic dysfunction occurs due to increased stiffness of the LV wall, which impairs diastolic blood flow from the left atrium to the left ventricle.

Echo Features of LV Diastolic Dysfunction

M-Mode MV Level

- Motion of the anterior mitral leaflet (AML) during normal diastole has a characteristic M-shape (E-A pattern). In the presence of LV diastolic dysfunction, AML excursion is diminished, A wave is taller than the E wave and the E:A ratio is reduced. These abnormalities are due to stiffness of the left ventricle and therefore greater atrial contribution towards ventricular filling. These signs are neither highly sensitive nor specific for the presence of diastolic dysfunction.

2-D Echo PLAX View

- 2-D echo cannot directly assess LV diastolic dysfunction. However, it can detect certain associated abnormalities such as ventricular hypertrophy, wall motion abnormality, myocardial infiltration or pericardial thickening.
- Coexistent abnormalities of LV systolic function may be detected.
- The diastolic flow pattern from the left atrium to the left ventricle can be assessed by pulsed wave (PW) Doppler using the apical 4-chamber view with the sample volume in the mitral inflow tract. This provides a good quality spectral tracing of mitral inflow velocity. In the normal heart, the transmitral flow pattern (Fig. 5.6A) shows the following waves:

  E wave   -   passive early diastolic LV filling
  A wave   -   active late diastolic LV filling
  E : A ratio   -   greater than 1

- When myocardial relaxation is impaired due to LV hypertrophy or myocardial ischemia, the A wave is large and E wave is small i.e. E:A ratio less than 1 (Fig. 5.6B). The deceleration time (DT) of the E wave is prolonged (> 220 msec). In persons aged > 50 yrs, the E : A ratio should be less than 0.5 to qualify for diastolic dysfunction since the A wave is already dominant at this age. This is known as the "slow-relaxation pattern" and indicates reduced LV compliance. There is increase in atrial dependent ventricular filling.

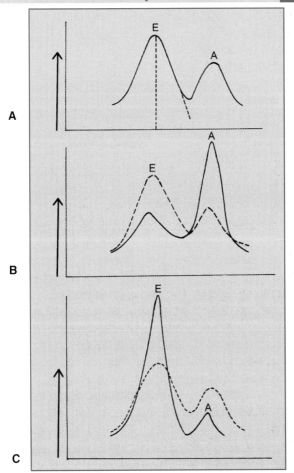

Fig. 5.6: The various patterns of mitral diastolic inflow seen on
PW doppler from the AP4CH view:
A. Normal flow pattern E > A,
B. Slow-relaxation pattern, A > E,
C. Restrictive pattern, very tall E

- When myocardial distensibility is impaired due to myocardial infiltration or pericardial constriction, the E wave is very tall and A wave is small (Fig. 5.6C). The deceleration time (DT) of the E wave is short (< 150 msec). This is known as the " restrictive pattern" and indicates an elevated LV end-diastolic pressure (LVEDP). All ventricular inflow occurs rapidly in early diastole and the atrium cannot distend the ventricle any further.

Pitfalls in the Diagnosis of LV Diastolic Dysfunction

- The mitral inflow pattern of LV filling is influenced by a large number of factors besides myocardial relaxation and distensibility. Therefore, it is inappropriate to rely only on E : A ratio as an indicator of LV diastolic dysfunction.
- Factors that influence the mitral inflow pattern include:
  — volume loading (preload and afterload)
  — heart rate and cardiac rhythm
  — left atrial systolic function
  — the phase of respiration
- Volume overloading due to mitral or aortic regurgitation attenuates the A wave since atrial contraction cannot effect forward flow if the ventricle is already maximally distended.
- In the presence of tachycardia, A wave is more prominent since the diastole is shortened (greater atrial contribution). When there is bradycardia, A wave is small since diastolic filling is prolonged (lesser atrial contribution). Therefore, a tall A wave is more significant in the presence of bradycardia.

- The E:A ratio is invalid in the presence of atrial fibrillation, complete heart block or a prolonged P-R interval.
- In an elderly person, the A wave is dominant. If the E:A ratio is >1 or E = A with short deceleration time (DT), it indicates the presence of an elevated LV end-diastolic pressure (LVEDP). This is referred to as pseudo-normalization of MV inflow pattern.

Causes of LV Diastolic Dysfunction

LV diastolic dysfunction is observed in the following conditions:
- Normal ageing (> 50 yrs)
- Left ventricular hypertrophy
- Coronary artery disease
- Restrictive cardiomyopathy
- Myocardial infiltration
- Pericardial constriction

Clinical Significance of LV diastolic Dysfunction

- The clinical features of left heart failure may occur in individuals with normal or near-normal LV systolic dysfunction as assessed by echo. These are often due to diastolic dysfunction.
- Diastolic dysfunction is observed in a variety of cardiac conditions. It is more sensitive than systolic dysfunction to the effects of normal ageing.
- Abnormalites of diastolic function may occur in isolation, may coexist with systolic dysfunction or may be observed before major systolic impairment

becomes obvious. Heart failure may be predominantly diastolic in one-third of the cases.

- LV systolic and diastolic function have to be assessed separately since their causation and more importantly their treatment is considerably different.

- Too simplistic a differentiation between diastolic and systolic dysfunction is often misleading. Systole and diastole are parts of a continuous cardiac cycle and interactions between them do occur. In mild systolic dysfunction with dyskinetic areas, some regions can continue contracting in diastole leading to shortening of the time available for ventricular filling. This leads to supervening diastolic dysfunction. Conversely, a poorly compliant left ventricle that fails to fill adequately in diastole may cause a low stroke volume in systole. This leads to supervening systolic dysfunction.

- Prominent A wave can be equated to the fourth heart sound (S4) on auscultation while a prominent E wave can be equated to the third heart sound (S3).

RV DYSFUNCTION

Whenever echocardiography is ordered or performed, the focus is always on the left ventricle. This is because the most common cardiac conditions namely systemic hypertension, coronary artery disease and mitral/aortic valvular pathologies affect the left ventricle. Nevertheless, the importance of the right ventricle and its role in heart disease is being increasingly recognized.

Normal Indices

RV internal dimension	7-23 mm
RV free-wall thickness	< 5 mm

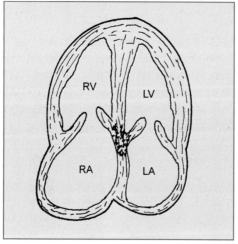

Fig. 5.7: Apical 4-chamber view showing dilatation of right atrium and right ventricle in a case of pulmonary hypertension

Echo Features of RV Dysfunction

- Right ventricular size and function can be evaluated by M-mode scan from the PLAX view and 2-D echo using the apical and subcostal 4- chamber views.
- RV dysfunction is associated with a dilated (> 23 mm) and hypokinetic RV. If the RV is of the same size or larger than the LV in all the echo-views, it is abnormal. An enlarged RV becomes globular and loses its normal triangular shape (Fig. 5.7).
- RV free-wall thickness > 5 mm is evidence of RV hypertrophy secondary to RV pressure overload as in pulmonary hypertension or pulmonary stenosis.
- Echo may reveal the underlying cause of RV dysfunction such as a left-to-right shunt or right-sided valvular disease.

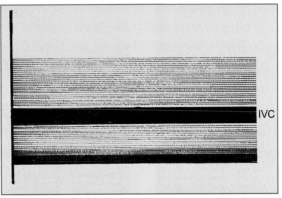

Fig. 5.8: Dilatation of the inferior vena cava (IVC)
beyond 2 cm in a case of right ventricular failure

- In the presence of RV failure, the right atrium is
  enlarged and the inferior vena cava is dilated beyond
  2 cm, which fails to constrict by atleast 50 percent
  during inspiration (Fig. 5.8).
- RV volume overload causes paradoxical motion of
  the interventricular septum (IVS) on M-mode scan
  from the parasternal long axis (PLAX) view.

Pitfalls in the Diagnosis of RV Dysfunction

- Echo assessment of the RV is difficult because of
  heavy trabeculation, its geometrical complexity and
  overlap with other chambers on imaging. Moreover,
  the RV is located directly under the sternum.
- Assessment of the RV is particularly difficult in the
  presence of lung hyperinflation (emphysema),
  pulmonary fibrosis and previous thoracic surgery.
  Paradoxically, study of RV function is all the more
  important in these subsets of patients.

- RV function is sensitive not only to myocardial contractility but also to loading conditions, LV contractility and septal excursion and to intrapericardial pressure. Analysis of RV function should take all these factors into account.
- Even in the most experienced hands, adequate echo examination of the RV is obtained in less than 50% of subjects.

Causes of RV Dysfunction

- Intracardiac left-to-right shunt—ASD, VSD.
- Right-sided valvular disease—TR, PR.
- Pulmonary hypertension—primary or secondary
- Right ventricular infarction—inferior wall MI
- Right ventricular dilatation—DCMP

Clinical Significance of RV Dysfunction

- Assessment of RV dysfunction plays a critical role in certain congenital and acquired cardiac conditions where it is important for planning treatment, timing surgical intervention and for predicting prognosis.
- In congenital heart disease such as VSD, ASD or Fallot's tetralogy, assessment of RV function before and after surgery is a useful prognostic marker.
- Similarly, timing of surgery in valvular heart disease such as MS, PS or TR is determined by the presence or absence of RV dysfunction.
- The long term prognosis of patients with chronic lung disease (COPD, ILD) depends upon RV function. RV dilatation, pulmonary hypertension and cor pulmonale carry a poor prognosis.

- Following myocardial infarction, RV dysfunction may be observed in the following 2 situations:
  a. inferior wall infarction with RV infarction.
  b. anterior wall infarction with acute VSD.

     RV infarction requires a different therapeutic approach than LV infarction. RV dysfunction due to post-MI VSD in an important cause of mortality (see Coronary Artery Disease).
- RV diastolic collapse is an important echo indicator of cardiac tamponade (see Pericardial Diseases).

CHAPTER SIX

CARDIOMYOPATHIES

The term cardiomyopathy means a disease of the heart muscle. In its strict sense, the term should only be applied to a condition that has no known underlying cause. In that case it known as an idiopathic cardio-myopathy. However, the term has through popular usage, been extended to include conditions where there is an identifiable cause. Examples of such conditions include hypertensive, ischemic, alcoholic and diabetic cardiomyopathy.

There are three important types of idiopathic cardio-myopathies.

1. Dilated cardiomyopathy   (DCMP)
2. Restrictive cardiomyopathy   (RCMP)
3. Hypertrophic cardiomyopathy   (HOCM)

DILATED CARDIOMYOPATHY (DCMP)

Echo Features of DCMP

M-Mode and 2-D Echo

- There is dilatation of all the four cardiac chambers particularly of the left ventricle, which thereby assumes a more globular shape (Fig. 6.1).
- Reduced LV wall thickness, reduced systolic thickening and reduced amplitude of wall motion. The reduced LV wall motion is generalized or global rather than regional. This is known as global hypokinesia. The LV walls are thin or there may be mild hypertrophy which is inadequate for the degree of LV dilatation.
- Left atrial enlargement occurs due to stretching of the mitral annular ring which leads to functional mitral regurgitation.

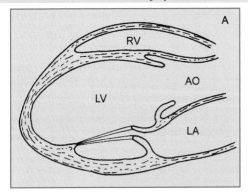

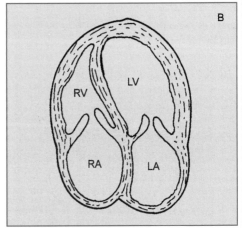

Fig. 6.1: Enlarged and globular-shaped left ventricle seen on PLAX view (A) and AP4CH view (B) in a patient with dilated cardiomyopathy

- Reduced motion of IVS and LVPW. Increased LVESD and LVEDD.

  Due to global hypokinesia, the systolic excursion of the interventricular septum and left ventricular posterior wall are reduced. For the same reason, the left ventricular diameter in end-diastole and end-systole is increased.

- Reduced fractional shortening (FS) and ejection fraction (LVEF). The ejection fraction (EF) is low but the cardiac output (CO) may be normal due to compensatory tachycardia. Due to global hypokinesia, indices of left ventricular systolic function are reduced (see Ventricular Function).

- Increased E-point septal separation (EPSS) (Fig. 6.2) This is the distance between the farthest posterior

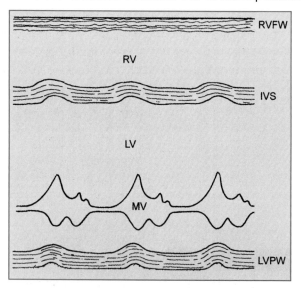

Fig. 6.2: M-mode scan from PLAX view showing:
     A dilated left ventricular cavity,
     B reduced movement of IVS and LVPW,
     C increased E-point septal separation,
     D reduced mitral leaflet excursion

excursion of the IVS and the E-point of the anterior mitral leaflet (AML). The normal EPSS does not exceed 5 mm.

Note: The EPSS is markedly reduced in hypertrophic cardiomyopathy (HOCM) due to systolic anterior motion (SAM) of anterior mitral leaflet (AML).

Measurement of EPSS is of no use in the presence of mitral valve disease which impairs free motion of the AML.

- Reduced anterior swing of aortic root during left atrial filling (normal > 7 mm)

Reduced AV cusp separation in systole (normal > 15 mm) with premature closure of the aortic valve (Fig. 6.3). Reduced MV anterior leaflet excursion in diastole (normal > 20 mm) with rapid upstroke and

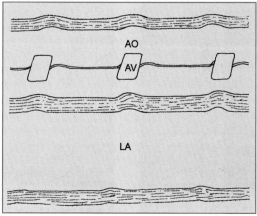

Fig. 6.3: M-mode scan from PLAX view at aortic valve level showing:
A Reduced aortic cusp separation,
B. Dilatation of the left atrium

downstroke. All the above are signs of reduced cardiac output.

- Associated non-specific findings in DCMP are:
  — small pericardial effusion
  — left ventricular thrombus

Doppler Echo

- Functional mitral and tricuspid regurgitation (MR and TR) occur due to stretching of atrio-ventricular (A-V) rings secondary to ventricular dilatation.

Differential Diagnosis of DCMP

It may be extremely difficult to differentiate dilated cardiomyopathy from the following conditions:
1. Severe MR with LV dysfunction
2. Ischemic cardiomyopathy (ICMP)

Severe MR with LV Dysfunction

Severe organic mitral regurgitation with volume overload and LV dysfunction can mimic DCMP with functional MR due to annular stretching. Organic MR with LV dysfunction is suggested if there is one of the following:
1. mitral leaflet thickening, prolapse or a flail leaflet
2. history of a long-standing pansystolic murmur.

Ischemic Cardiomyopathy (ICMP)

DCMP can closely mimic ICMP with the following subtle differences (Table 6.1):
1. in DCMP there is global hypokinesia while in ICMP, atleast one region of the left ventricle moves normally.

Table 6.1: Differences between dilated and ischemic cardiomyopathy		
	DCMP	*ICMP*
Hypokinesia	Global	Regional
RWMA and arterial territory	Do not conform	Conform
Dyskinesia	Not seen	Seen
RV involvement	Often	Rare

2. in DCMP if there is patchy involvement, the regional wall motion abnormalities (RWMAs) do not conform to arterial distribution. On the other hand in ICMP, RWMAs conform to coronary territories.
3. right ventricle is often involved in DCMP but relatively spared in ICMP.
4. dyskinetic areas and aneurysms are a feature of ICMP and not DCMP.

Causes of DCMP

- Idiopathic
- Post-viral
- Alcoholic
- Diabetic
- Peripartum
- Drug-induced
- Nutritional

Causes of Large LV in Infancy

- Congenital cardiomyopathy
- Coarctation of aorta
- Anomalous left coronary artery arising from pulmonary artery (ALCAPA)

RESTRICTIVE CARDIOMYOPATHY (RCMP)

Echo Features of RCMP

M-mode and 2-D echo

- Thickening of LV and RV free wall and IVseptum. The thickness of LVPW and IVS in diastole exceeds 12 mm and that of the RV free wall is >5 mm.
- Bright echogenicity of endocardium with patches of speckling or mottling in the myocardium. Infiltration of amyloid into the IV septum produces a sparkling 'ground-glass' appearance.
- Reduced internal dimensions and cavity size of LV and RV with cavity obliteration at LV and RV apex (Fig. 6.4).

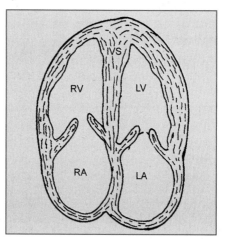

Fig. 6.4: Apical 4-chamber view showing:
A. Thickening of IV septum,
B. Reduction of RV and LV size and obliteration of RV and LV apex in a case of restrictive cardiomyopathy

- Mild impairment of LV systolic function with reduced IVS and LVPW thickening and inward motion during systole
- Thickening of MV and TV leaflets
- Dilated right and left atrium.
- Small pericardial effusion.
- Ventricular mural thrombus.

Doppler Echo

- Mitral and tricuspid regurgitation (MR and TR) due to thickening of MV and TV leaflets.
- Impairment of LV and RV diastolic function with a slow relaxation pattern (A taller than E) or a restrictive pattern (very tall E) seen on MV inflow spectral tracing (Fig. 6.5).

Differential Diagnosis of RCMP

- It may be extremely difficult to differentiate restrictive cardiomyopathy from constrictive pericarditis on the basis of echo findings. Often cardiac catheterization

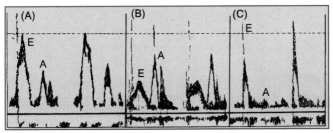

Fig. 6.5: Different patterns of mitral diastolic inflow seen on PW Doppler tracing:
A. Normal flow pattern. E > A,
B. Slow-relaxation pattern. A > E,
C. Restrictive pattern. Very tall E

is required for this purpose. The differentiation between the two conditions is important as it has crucial management implications. The following features are observed only in RCMP and not in constrictive pericarditis:

thickening of ventricular walls.
reduction of ventricular cavity size
mild impairment of LV systolic function
mitral and tricuspid regurgitation
dilatation of right and left atrium
(see Pericardial Diseases)

- RCMP needs to be differentiated from apical cardio-myopathy, a sub-type of hypertrophic cardiomyopathy, where the hypertrophy is confined to the apices of the ventricles with obliteration of ventricular cavity. In both these condition, the right and left atrium are enlarged. The only other cardiac condition in which both the atria are enlarged with normal or small ventricles is mitral stenosis with pulmonary hyper-tension and secondary tricuspid regurgitation. In dilated cardiomyopathy there is enlargement of all the four cardiac chambers.

Causes of RCMP

- Idiopathic
- Endomyocardial fibrosis (EMF)
- Myocardial infiltration due to
    amyloidosis
    sarcoidosis
    malignancy
    haemochromatosis
    glycogen storage diseases

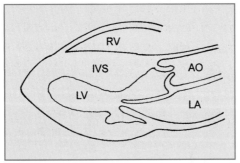

Fig. 6.6: Parasternal long-axis view showing asymmetrical septal hypertrophy (ASH) of the interventricular septum (IVS) in a case of HOCM

HYPERTROPHIC CARDIOMYOPATHY (HOCM)

Echo Features of HOCM

M-mode and 2-D Echo

- Asymmetrical septal hypertrophy (ASH). There is hypertrophy of the interventricular septum (IVS) to a greater extent than that of the LV posterior wall (LVPW) (Fig. 6.6). An IVS : LVPW ratio of 1.5 or more is unequivocal evidence of ASH. The thickness of IVS and LVPW in diastole exceeds 12 mm.
- ASH is observed in 60% cases of HOCM while 30% show concentric myocardial hypertrophy and in 5-10% cases, the hypertrophy is confined to the apices of the ventricles i.e. apical cardiomyopathy (Fig. 6.7).
- The thickened IVS shows bright echogenicity with speckling in the myocardium due to myocardial fibre disarray. Thickening of the IV septum is confined to the base and impinges on the LV outflow tract.

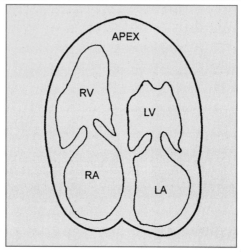

Fig. 6.7: Apical 4-chamber view showing hypertrophy confined to the left ventricular apex in a case of apical cardiomyopathy

- There is reduced IVS motion with vigorous excursion of the LV posterior wall (LVPW). The LV cavity appears smaller in volume than normal.
- Systolic anterior motion (SAM) of anterior mitral leaflet (AML) (Fig. 6.8). During later part of systole, the AML moves anteriorly to coapt with the IVS. This occurs due to Venturi effect caused by high velocity in the LV outflow tract (LVOT). SAM occurs during later stage of systole when the LV cavity size becomes smaller. SAM causes dynamic LVOT obstruction. Thus the term hypertrophic obstructive cardiomyopathy (HOCM) is more appropriate. If no LVOT obstruction is demonstrable, the terminology used is non-obstructive idiopathic hypertrophic sub-aortic stenosis (IHSS).

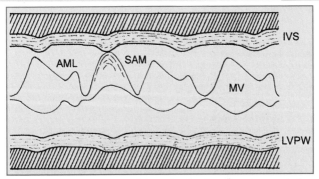

Fig. 6.8: M-mode scan of the mitral valve showing systolic anterior motion (SAM) of anterior mitral leaflet (AML)

- LVOT obstruction may be present at rest or become more pronounced following provocation. Provocation may be provided by prolonged standing, isovolumic exercise (e.g. hand-grip), Valsalva manoeuvre or sublingual nitrate. All these methods reduce LV size and thus increase the likelihood of LVOT obstruction.
- Dynamic LVOT obstruction during later part of systole causes mid-systolic aortic valve closure and late-systolic aortic cusp fluttering (Fig. 6.9).

Doppler Echo

- On CW Doppler, there is increased peak flow velocity across the LVOT. PW Doppler with the sample volume in the LVOT shows the increased velocity to be proximal to the aortic valve. The high velocity jet has a characteristic concave appearance with the peak velocity (Vmax) coinciding with peak SAM and most of aortic flow occurring prior to Vmax (Fig. 6.10).

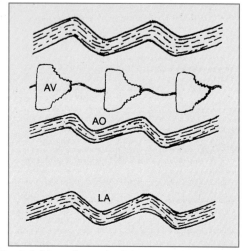

Fig. 6.9: M-mode scan of the aortic valve showing mid-systolic closure and late-systolic fluttering

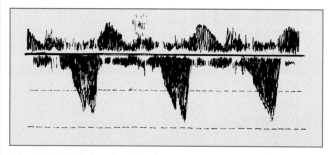

Fig. 6.10: CW doppler showing a concave high velocity jet in the LV outflow tract, proximal to the aortic valve

- There are features of LV diastolic dysfunction due to myocardial hypertrophy with an abnormal transmitral inflow spectral trace – A wave taller than E (see Ventricular Dysfunction).

- Mitral regurgitation is frequently associated with LVOT obstruction.

Differential Diagnosis of HOCM

- An IVS : LVPW ratio of 1.5 or more is evidence of ASH of HOCM.
  A ratio of 1.3 to 1.5 may be observed in :
    Hypertension with LVH
    Aortic stenosis with LVH
    Septal infiltration (RCMP)
- Localized subaortic bulging of the IV septum is a normal finding in the elderly and should not be misdiagnosed as HOCM.
- Reduced IVS motion with vigorous LVPW excursion is a feature of HOCM. Reduced IVS motion is also observed in DCMP and old myocardial infarction with the following differences:
    in DCMP, the LVPW is also hypokinetic like the IV septum
    in old septal MI, the LVPW shows compensatory hyperkinesia
- Systolic anterior motion (SAM) of the anterior mitral leaflet (AML) is also observed in:
  Mitral valve prolapse (anterior buckling of AML)
  Hyperdynamic circulation (vigorous cardiac systolic excursion)
  Pericardial effusion (pseudo-SAM during anterior swing).
- Mid-systolic aortic valve closure occurs in HOCM due to dynamic LVOT obstruction. Mid-systolic AV closure is also observed in :

subvalvular aortic stenosis
MR (LV ejection into LA)
VSD (LV ejection into RV)

- The peak flow velocity across the LVOT in HOCM can be differentiated from valvular aortic stenosis by the following features :
  on PW Doppler the Vmax is proximal to the AV
  the flow velocity jet has a typical concave pattern.
- LV diastolic dysfunction in HOCM can be differentiated from that due to RCMP by the presence of ASH, SAM, LVOT obstruction and early AV closure
- The high velocity jet across LVOT in HOCM needs to be differentiated from the adjacent jet of mitral regurgitation which is frequently coexistent. The timing and concave appearance of the HOCM jet are differentiating features.

CHAPTER SEVEN

CORONARY ARTERY DISEASE

Since coronary artery disease (CAD) is the leading form of heart disease in middle and old ages, it is therefore not surprising that CAD is the commonest clinical diagnosis in those on whom echo is performed.

INDICATIONS FOR ECHO IN CAD

- Detection and assessment of extent of myocardial ischemia.
- Detection and assessment of extent of myocardial infarction.
- Assessment of left ventricular diastolic and systolic function.
- Detection of right ventricular infarction and dysfunction.
- Detection of the complications of acute myocardial infarction
  — acute mitral regurgitation
  — acute ventricular septal defect
  — ventricular aneurysm
  — pericardial effusion
  — mural thrombus.
- Direct visualization of coronary arteries for anomalies
  — proximal coronary stenosis
  — coronary artery aneurysm
  — coronary artery fistula
  — anomalous origin of artery
- Diagnosis of cardiac conditions simulating CAD.
  — aortic stenosis (AS)
  — MV prolapse (MVP)
  — hypertrophic CMP (HOCM)
- Stress echocardiography (post-exercise echo)

— if TMT is not possible, uninterpretable or equivocal.
— to localize the site and quantify extent of ischemia
— to assess myocardial viability:stunning or hibernation.

MYOCARDIAL ISCHEMIA

- Abnormal systolic wall thickening: reduced or absent. Thickening of the ischemic myocardial segment during systole is reduced in extent or altogether absent.
- Abnormal systolic wall motion: hypokinesia, akinesia or dyskinesia.
  Inward motion of the ischemic myocardial segment during systole is reduced, absent or paradoxically outwards.
- These changes are reversible if ischemia is reversed by rest or giving nitrates. Acute myocardial infarction causes similar abnormalities which are reversible by thrombolytic therapy or primary angioplasty. Abnormal wall motion can be classified as below, with each pattern of wall motion assigned a score:
  1. normal motion   full inward motion
  2. hypokinesia   < 50% inward motion
  3. akinesia   no inward motion
  4. dyskinesia   outward movement
  5. aneurysmal   outpouching of wall.
- From the wall motion score, the wall motion index can be calculated as follows:

$$\text{Wall motion index} = \frac{\text{sum of scores of all segments}}{\text{number of segments studied}}$$

A wall motion index more than 1.5 is significant.

MYOCARDIAL INFARCTION

- Abnormal systolic wall thickening: reduced or absent. Thickening of the infarcted myocardial segment during systole is reduced in extent or altogether absent. There may be actual systolic thinning to < 7 mm or by >30% compared to the adjacent myocardium, if the infarct is old.
- The thinned myocardial scar is more echoreflective than the adjacent myocardium, due to post-infarction fibrosis
- Abnormal systolic wall motion: hypokinesia, akinesia or dyskinesia

  Inward motion of the infarcted myocardial segment during systole is reduced, absent or paradoxically outwards (Fig. 7.1).

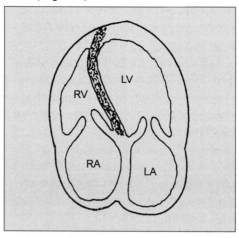

Fig. 7.1: Apical 4-chamber view showing a thinned out and scarred myocardial segment that moves paradoxically outwards during systole

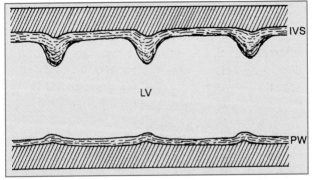

Fig. 7.2: M-mode scan at the ventricular level showing hypo-kinesia of the posterior wall with compensatory hyperkinesia of the interventricular septum

Dyskinetic segments and aneurysmal areas are more often due to old myocardial infarction than due to ischemia, because of prior myocardial scarring. Wall motion abnormalities due to infarction are not reversible by rest or giving nitrates.

- The normal myocardial segment facing the wall that shows abnormal motion may show compensatory hyperkinesia and exaggerated contraction (Fig. 7.2).

The areas of the left ventricle which can be studied from several echo views are:

IV septum (Fig. 7.3)
ventricular apex (Fig. 7.4)
anterior wall (Fig. 7.5)
lateral wall (Fig. 7.6)
inferior wall. (Fig. 7.7)

On 2-D imaging, the left ventricle can be divided up into several segments. This is useful to localize the site of ischemia /infarction and to quantify its extent. Each

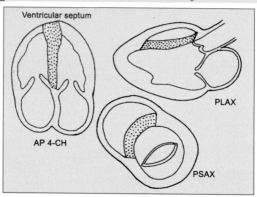

Ventricular septum

AP 4-CH

PLAX

PSAX

Fig. 7.3

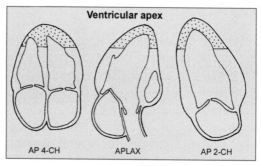

Ventricular apex

AP 4-CH   APLAX   AP 2-CH

Fig. 7.4

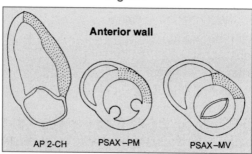

Anterior wall

AP 2-CH   PSAX –PM   PSAX –MV

Fig. 7.5

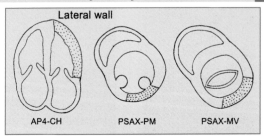

Fig. 7.6

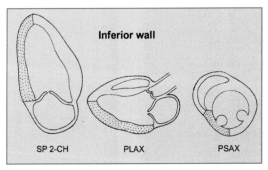

Fig. 7.7

wall can be further divided into basal (proximal), mid and apical (distal) segments.

From the location pattern of wall motion abnormalities, it is possible to predict the coronary artery that is involved (Fig. 7.8).

LEFT VENTRICULAR DYSFUNCTION

• Presence of coronary artery disease ever without prior myocardial infarction can cause LV diastolic dysfunction (impaired myocardial relaxation).

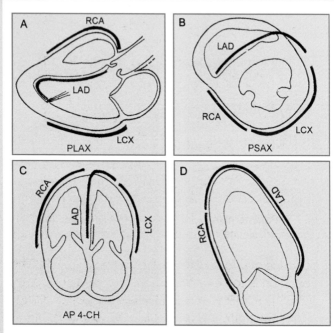

Fig. 7.8: The arterial supply of the heart:
A   PLAX view   LAD : Left anterior descending
B   PSAX view   LCX : Left circumflex artery
C   AP4CH view   RCA : Right coronary artery
D   AP2CH view

- A single large myocardial infarction or repeated small infarcts leads to scarring of myocardium resulting in thin segments which do not thicken during systole and show abnormal motion. This is often associated with LV systolic dysfunction.
- Triple vessel coronary artery disease may lead to impairment of LV systolic dysfunction even in the

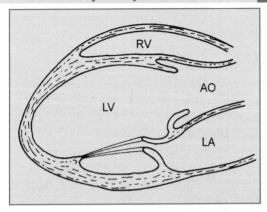

Fig. 7.9: Parasternal long-axis view showing enlargement of the left ventricular cavity in a case of ischemic cardiomyopathy

absence of prior myocardial infarction (Fig. 7.9). This condition is referred to as ischemic cardiomyopathy (ICMP). ICMP superficially resembles a dilated cardiomyopathy (DCMP) with the following subtle differences:

1. in ICMP, atleast one portion of the LV moves normally while global hypokinesia is often observed in DCMP.
2. dyskinetic areas and aneurysms are a feature of ICMP and not DCMP.
3. in ICMP wall motion abnormalities conform to specific arterial territories.
4. the right ventricle is usually spared in ICMP and often involved in DCMP. (see Cardiomyopathies).

- Following temporary coronary occlusion, impairment of myocardial contractile function may remain, even after restoration of blood supply without infarction. This is termed as myocardial stunning and the myocardial tissue remains viable to regain normal function after 1 to 2 weeks. Similarly, recurrent episodes of acute ischemia may result in temporary myocardial dysfunction which is termed as myocardial hibernation. Myocardium that is stunned or hibernating does not have enough energy to contract but is still viable and able to repair wear and tear. A stunned or hibernating myocardium may cause LV systolic or diastolic dysfunction which is reversible by revascularization.

- Cardiogenic shock after acute myocardial infarction may be due to pump failure following extensive muscle damage. In this condition, echo shows severe impairment of LV systolic function. Alternatively, it may be due to LV free wall rupture, haemopericardium and cardiac tamponade. In acute mitral regurgitation or acute ventricular septal defect after myocardial infarction, LV systolic function remains active.

RIGHT VENTRICULAR DYSFUNCTION

- Whenever echocardiography is performed for assessment of coronary artery disease, the focus is on the left ventricle. Nevertheless, evaluation of the right ventricle is important, particularly in patients of inferior wall infarction. In them, prognosis is worse if there is right ventricular infarction and RV dysfunction.

- The haemodynamic response of the right ventricle to myocardial infarction is different from that of the left ventricle. When there is RV infarction, cardiogenic shock is common and it requires a different therapeutic approach than does LV infarction (saline infusion

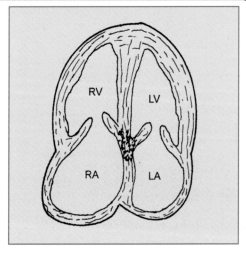

Fig. 7.10: Apical 4-chamber view showing dilatation of the right ventricle and right atrium in a case of right ventricular infarction

and not diuresis). It is suspected clinically by the presence of hypotension with a raised jugular venous pressure (JVP)

- RV infarction is associated with a dilated (> 23 mm) and hypokinetic right ventricle. There is paradoxical motion of the IV septum. The right atrium is dilated (Fig. 7.10). Due to RV failure, the inferior vena cava (IVC) is dilated beyond 2cm and fails to constrict by atleast 50% during inspiration.
- Evaluation of RV function is also useful in assessing the prognosis of patients with ventricular septal defect (acute VSD) following myocardial infarction. RV dysfunction is a predictor of cardiogenic shock and mortality in these patients.

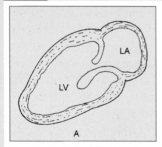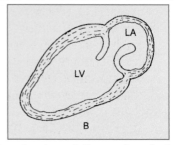

Fig. 7.11: Apical 2-chamber view showing a flail posterior mitral leaflet showing exaggerated motion from:

A. Left ventricle in diastole to

B. Left atrium in systole

ACUTE MITRAL REGURGITATION

- Acute MR in a setting of acute myocardial infarction occurs either due to papillary muscle rupture or because of papillary muscle dysfunction.

- Rupture of a papillary muscle causes a flail mitral valve leaflet. Since rupture of the postero-medial papillary muscle is more common than that of the antero-lateral muscle, often it is the posterior mitral leaflet (PML) that is flail. It generally follows inferior wall infarction due to occlusion of the posterior descending branch of the right coronary artery.

- On 2-D Echo, the flail leaflet exhibits an exaggerated whip-like motion (like a sail flapping in the wind). Its tip moves past the coaptation point into the left atrium and fails to coapt with the AML (Fig. 7.11). Superficially, it resembles the floppy leaflet of mitral valve prolapse (see Valvular Diseases).

- Papillary muscle dysfunction is due to ischemic restriction of papillary function or akinesia of the infero-basal wall that does not shorten in systole. As a result, the posterior MV leaflet fails to reach the plane of the MV annulus and the AML/PML coaptation point in systole is distally located in the left ventricle.

- On continuous wave (CW) Doppler or colour flow mapping, the MR flow velocity or colour jet is eccentric and directed towards the posterior left atrial wall. The jet area may be much less than what the actual amount of MR would indicate hence there is a risk of underestimation of MR severity.
- Unlike in the MR of valvular disease, in acute MR there is no dilatation of the left atrium and ventricle or abnormal architecture of the MV leaflets.
- In acute MR due to acute MI, LV systolic function remains active unlike in pump failure due to extensive MI in which case there is severe LV impairment.

ACUTE VENTRICULAR SEPTAL DEFECT

- Ventricular septal defect (acquired VSD) in a setting of acute myocardial infarction occurs due to a breach in continuity of the interventricular septum. It often occurs near the cardiac apex and is more common after damage to the inferior wall with right ventricular infarction.
- The discontinuity in the IV septum can be seen as an echo dropout on 2-D echo in several views. The perforation expands in systole and often there is an aneurysmal bulge of the septum close to the LV apex.
- The VSD jet can be seen on colour flow mapping and by moving the pulsed wave (PW) Doppler along the RV side of the septum on the PLAX and AP4CH views (Fig. 7.12).

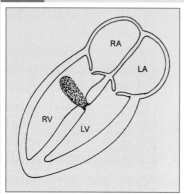

Fig. 7.12: Illustrative diagram showing a high velocity jet across a ventricular septal defect, on Doppler echo

- Significant left-to-right shunting of blood across the VSD can cause RV volume overload. As in acute MR, the LV systolic function remains active in acute VSD.

LEFT VENTRICULAR ANEURYSM

- An aneurysm is a large bulge-like deformity with a wide neck, located at or near the apex of the left ventricle. It is more common after damage to the anterior wall than after inferior wall infarction. The aneurysm exhibits dyskinesia or outward systolic expansion and a persistent diastolic deformity (Fig. 7.13). The wall of the aneurysm is made of myocardium and is more echogenic than adjacent areas because of fibrous scar tissue. It does not rupture but is often associated with a pedunculated or laminated ventricular thrombus.
- A false aneurysm (pseudo-aneurysm) follows a breach in the left ventricular free wall, when the resulting haemopericardium clots and seals off the

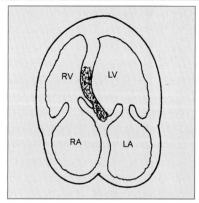

Fig. 7.13: Apical 4-chamber view showing an aneurysmal bulge in the basal portion of interventricular septum

hole in the wall by pericardial adhesions. The neck of the pseudo-aneurysm that communicates with the left ventricle is narrower than the diameter of the aneurysm. Therefore, it appears as a globular extracardiac pouch, external to the LV cavity. A false aneurysm is located on the posterolateral LV wall and is more common after inferior wall than after anterior wall infarction. It is non-expansile and remains constant in size. The wall of the aneurysm is made of pericardium and it is less echogenic than adjacent areas. It is friable, liable to rupture and is often filled with a thrombus due to clotted haemopericardium.

- The differences between a true and false LV aneurysm are enumerated in Table 7.1.

VENTRICULAR MURAL THROMBUS

- A ventricular thrombus may form on a dyskinetic, infarcted and scarred myocardial segment or within a left ventricular aneurysm.

Table 7.1: Differences between true LV aneurysm and pseudo-aneurysm

	LV aneurysm	*Pseudo-aneurysm*
Shape	Wide neck	Narrow neck
Location	Apex of LV	Posterior wall
Expansion	Outward in systole	Non-expansile
Wall	Myocardium	Pericardium
Rupture	Unlikely	Liable
Thrombus	Mobile/laminated	Fills cavity

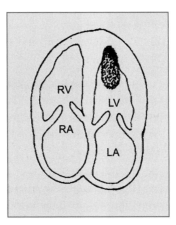

Fig. 7.14: Apical 4-chamber view showing a left ventricular thrombus protruding into the LV cavity

- It appears as a rounded pedunculated mass protruding into the LV cavity (Fig. 7.14) or as a flat laminated mural thrombus contiguous with the ventricular wall.
- A mobile mural thrombus may be a source of peripheral embolization (see Intracardiac Masses)

ACUTE PERICARDIAL EFFUSION

- A small amount of pericardial effusion may accumulate due to pericardial reaction to transmural myocardial infarction.
- A rupture of the left ventricular free wall may lead to haemopericardium. This may cause cardiac tamponade which is usually rapidly fatal.
- Sometimes the haemopericardium clots, seals off the hole by adhesions and forms a pseudo-aneurysm (see above).
- An auto-immune pericarditis with a small amount of effusion may follow acute myocardiac infarction. This is known as the Dressler's syndrome.

CORONARY ARTERY ANOMALIES

Echocardiography is not the best investigative modality to visualize abnormalities of the coronary arterial tree. Coronary angiography is the best investigation for this purpose. Rarely, direct visualization of the coronary arteries may reveal the following abnormalites:

1. Proximal coronary stenosis seen as focal reduction in lumen size or focal increase in reflectivity of the proximal 1.0-1.5 cm of the coronary artery.
2. Coronary artery aneurysm seen as a circular echo-free space e.g. Kawasaki syndrome
3. Coronary artery fistula seen as parallel echoes with a wide lumen.
4. Anomalous origin of artery seen as a dilated right coronary artery with left coronary artery arising from the pulmonary artery. This condition is known as

ALCAPA (anomalous left coronary artery arising from pulmonary artery.)

SIMULATING CONDITIONS

The commonest form of coronary artery disease is narrowing of the vessel lumen by atherosclerotic plaque(s). The most frequent symptom of CAD is chest pain (angina pectoris) due to myocardial ischemia. This anginal pain needs to be differentiated from other causes of chest pain such as oesophageal disorders and musculoskeletal diseases. Occasionally, the chest pain is caused by cardiac conditions that simulate CAD in their clinical presentation. These conditions can be readily diagnosed by echocardiography and they include:

1. Aortic valve stenosis (AS)
2. Mitral valve prolapse (MVP)
3. Hypertrophic CMP (HOCM)

STRESS ECHOCARDIOGRAPHY

Principle

Stress echo is a technique to demonstrate abnormalities of regional wall motion and thickening which are not present when an echo is performed at rest. In other words, it picks up inducible or provokable ischemia in response to stress.

Method

The stress is delivered by one of the following methods:

1. Physical exercise (treadmill or bicycle) as used for exercise stress ECG testing
2. Pharmacological stress using dobutamine (vasodilating inotropic agent) or adenosine (vasodilator that diverts blood away from area served by stenotic artery.)
3. Cardiac pacing (to increase heart rate and thus simulate exercise).

Indications

1. As an alternative to stress ECG testing in the following situations:
   a. inability to exercise on a treadmill / bicycle.
   b. resting ECG abnormality (LBBB, LVH, digoxin)
   c. equivocal or inconclusive stress ECG testing.
   The sensitivity and specificity of stress echocardiography for detection of coronary disease (80% and 90% respectively), is higher than that of stress ECG testing (65% and 75% respectively). It is quite similar to that of radionuclide myocardial perfusion imaging (stress thallium). Wall motion abnormalities occur earlier than either chest pain or ST segment changes of ischemia.
2. To localize the site and to quantify extent of ischemia
   As mentioned under myocardial infarction, the left ventricle can be divided up into several segments to study wall motion abnormalities. From the pattern of abnormal motion, not only can ischemia be quantified but also the occluded coronary artery can be predicted. This is helpful in the following situations:

a. to select patients for early coronary angiography and revascularization e.g. large wall motion abnormality in LAD territory.
b. to stratify the risk of a future coronary event after acute myocardial infarction.
c. to assess the functional significance of a known stenotic lesion while planning angioplasty or by-pass surgery.

3. To assess myocardial viability—stunning or hibernation

Myocardium that is stunned or hibernating causes LV systolic or diastolic dysfunction which is reversible by revascularization. If hibernation is present but the heart is not revascularized, mortality is far higher than if there is no viability at all. This fact underscores the importance of detecting hibernating myocardium. Stress echo is similar in sensitivity to position emission tomography (PET) for detection of myocardial viability.

Positivity

The stress echo test is considered positive in the following situations :
1. worsening of previous wall motion abnormality.
2. appearance of new wall motion abnormality
3. failure to rise or fall in ejection fraction
4. appearance or worsening of mitral regurgitation

Limitations

1. high degree of operator dependancy
2. difficult acoustic windows in presence of obesity or emphysema

3. unclear imaging during post-exercise heavy breathing.

4. difficulty in delineation of the endocardial lining leading to error in volumetric measurement.

5. presence of septal dyskinesia due to left bundle branch block.

6. False negative test in the following situations:
   a. small ischemic area with good collateralization
   b. single vessel disease without prior infarction.
   c. operator inexperience, heavy breathing,
   d. difficult window, post-exercise time-lag

CHAPTER EIGHT

SYSTEMIC HYPERTENSION

Since systemic hypertension is a common clinical condition, echo is often performed in hypertensive subjects.

Indications for Echo in Hypertension

- Detection of left ventricular hypertrophy (LVH) (see below)
- Assessment of LV systolic and diastolic dysfunction (see Ventricular Dysfunction)
- Detection of coexisting coronary artery disease (CAD) (see Coronary Artery Disease)
- Detection of mitral and aortic valve degeneration (see Valvular Diseases)
- Detection of aortic dilatation and coarctation (see Aortic Diseases)

Echo Features of LV Hypertrophy

- Thickening of the interventricular septum (IVS) and left ventricular posterior wall (LVPW). The normal thickness of the IVS and LVPW in diastole is 6 to 12 mm. Thickness exceeding 12 mm indicates the presence of left ventricular hypertrophy (LVH) (Fig. 8.1).
- Normally the ratio of IVS : LVPW thickness is 1:1. Hypertrophy of the IVS to a greater extent than that of the LVPW indicates asymmetrical septal hypertrophy (ASH). If there is ASH in hypertension, the IVS : LVPW ratio is usually in the range of 1.3 to 1.5.
- Small left ventricular cavity. Thickening of the IVS and LVPW leads to obliteration of the LV cavity in systole since the LV systolic function is usually good and the amplitude of wall motion is normal. Thick papillary

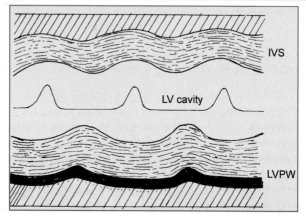

Fig. 8.1: M-mode scan at ventricular level showing marked thickening of the IV septum and LV posterior wall with obliteration of LV cavity. This patient has concentric LVH due to long-standing systemic hypertension

muscles with prominent trabeculae carnae are seen parallel to the LV posterior wall.

- There is an increase in the left ventricular mass. The LV mass in grams is calculated by the following equation:

LV mass =

$$1.04 [(IVS + LVPW + LVEDD)^3 - LVEDD^3] - 14$$

IVS is diastolic thickness of IV septum
LVPW is diastolic thickness of posterior wall
LVEDD is end-diastolic dimension of ventricle.

LV mass can also be calculated by subtracting LV endocardial volume (LVV endo) from the LV epicardial volume (LVV epi) and multiplying it by the density of the muscle which is 1.055 g/cm^3. This is because mass is the product of volume and density.

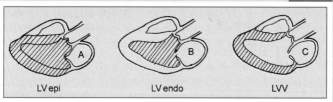

Fig. 8.2: Calculation of left ventricular mass from LV volume. LV volume (C) = LV epicardial volume (A) minus LV endocardial volume (B)

LV mass = [LVVepi - LVV endo] × 1.055 (Fig. 8.2)
In the presence of LV hypertrophy, the LV mass exceeds 134 grams in men and 110 grams in women per meter square body surface area.

- In LV hypertrophy due to hypertension the increase in wall thickness occurs at the expense of reduction in cavity size. This is known as concentric LVH. In concentric LVH, the relative wall thickness (RWT) ratio, which is LVPW thickness divided by LV radius in diastole, exceeds 0.45.

Differential Diagnosis of Hypertensive LVH

- The echo picture of LVH due to hypertension is simulated by LVH due to other conditions causing LV pressure overload namely aortic valve stenosis and coarctation of aorta.
- The asymmetrical septal hypertrophy (ASH) in hypertension may resemble ASH due to hypertrophic cardiomyopathy (HOCM). However, the IVS : LVPW ratio in hypertension is generally in the range of 1.3 to 1.5 while it exceeds 1.5 in HOCM.
- Myocardial thickening with LV diastolic dysfunction is also observed in restrictive cardiomyopathy

(RCMP) and myocardial infiltrative diseases. These can be differentiated from the effects of systemic hypertension by the lack of coexisting coronary arterial, valvular and aortic abnormalities and an absent history of hypertension.

- Systemic hypertension, aortic stenosis and coarctation of aorta cause LV pressure overload. Mitral and aortic regurgitation, chronic anaemia and chronic renal failure cause LV volume overload. In conditions causing LV volume overload, there is predominant LV dilatation with a mild degree of LVH. In these conditions there is eccentric LVH which is inadequate for the degree of LV dilatation. The relative wall thickness (RWT) ratio, which is LVPW thickness divided by LV radius in diastole, is less than 0.45.

- In eccentric LV hypertrophy the degree of LVH, as determined only from wall thickness, may be underestimated. However, even in this condition the left ventricular muscle mass is increased. Therefore, LV muscle mass is a better indicator of LV hypertrophy than LV wall thickness.

- In the advanced stages of hypertensive heart disease, there is LV dilatation, global hypokinesia and LV systolic dysfunction. The echo picture then resembles that of dilated cardiomyopathy (DCMP). This underscores the importance of serial echos in evaluation of the effects of systemic hypertension on the left ventricle.

Clinical Significance of LVH in Hypertension

- Presence of LVH is the most common abnormality on echo in a hypertensive patient. Systemic hypertension is also the most important cause of LVH.

- LVH is an independent predictor of cardiovascular morbidity and mortality as a risk factor for myocardial infarction, heart failure and sudden cardiac death. The predictive value of LVH in hypertension is as strong as that of multi-vessel coronary artery disease.

- LVH may be indicated on the ECG by presence of tall QRS complexes. The voltage criteria of S in V_1 or V_2 plus R in V_5 or V_6 greater than 35 mm (Sokolow criteria) is often used. There may be an associated 'strain pattern' with ST segment depression and T wave inversion in the lateral leads. Echocardiography is 5 to 10 times more sensitive than ECG at detecting LVH.

- Presence of LVH can be used as an indication for treatment of young patients having borderline or labile hypertension. In them, echo is also useful to screen for an underlying coarctation of aorta.

- Serial echos may be performed periodically (e.g. annually) to monitor the progress of hypertensive heart disease and to assess the regression of LVH with antihypertensive drugs.

CHAPTER NINE

PULMONARY HYPERTENSION

Normal Indices

RV internal dimension	< 23 mm
RV free-wall thickness	< 5 mm
Pulmonary artery width	= aortic width.
Pulmonary artery pressure	< 25 mm Hg.

Echo Features of Pulmonary Hypertension

M-mode PV Level

- The pulmonary valve leaflet shows flattening or loss of the normal presystolic 'a' wave. Due to high pulmonary artery pressure, right atrial contraction in pre-systole has no effect on the pulmonary valve.
- There is a mid-systolic notch due to brief closure of the pulmonary valve, followed by reopening in late-systole (Fig. 9.1).
- The ratio between pre-ejection period (PEP) and right ventricular ejection time (RVET) exceeds 0.4. This is due to prolonged isovolumic RV contraction

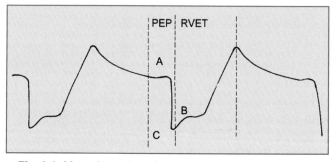

Fig. 9.1: M-mode tracing of the pulmonary leaflet showing:
A. flattening of the 'a' wave,
B. a mid-systolic notch,
C. Prolonged pre-ejection period (PEP). RVET is right ventricular ejection time

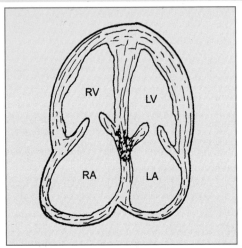

Fig. 9.2: Apical 4-chamber view showing dilatation
of the right atrium and right ventricle

(RV pressure takes longer to exceed the raised PA
pressure)

2-D Echo PLAX and PSAX Views

- There is dilatation of the right ventricle > 23 mm with
  or without RV hypertrophy i.e. free wall thickness
  > 5 mm in the PLAX view (Fig. 9.2).
- Paradoxical motion of interventricular septum (IVS)
  is observed. The IVS moves away from the left
  ventricle and towards the right ventricle in systole. It
  seems to be a part of the right ventricle which here
  has a greater stroke volume than the left ventricle.
- In the PSAX view at the level of the aortic valve, the
  diameter of the pulmonary artery exceeds the width
  of the aorta.

- The underlying cause of pulmonary hypertension such as mitral stenosis or a septal defect may be picked up.

Doppler Echo

- A jet of pulmonary regurgitation (PR) may be observed in the right ventricular outflow tract (RVOT) on colour flow mapping. On PW Doppler, a high velocity signal is picked up just below the pulmonary valve.

Doppler Calculations

- The pulmonary artery pressure can be measured from the peak transtricuspid flow velocity (Vmax). This is obtained by Doppler spectral display of tricuspid regurgitant jet in the apical 4-chamber view (Fig. 9.3).

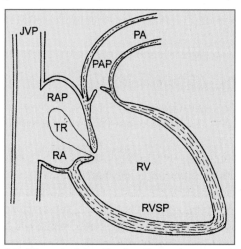

Fig. 9.3: The principle of estimating pulmonary artery pressure from the tricuspid regurgitant jet

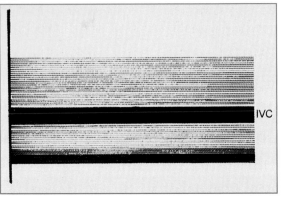

Fig. 9.4: Dilatation of the inferior vena cava (IVC) beyond 2 cm in a case of pulmonary hypertension

Pulsed wave (PW) Doppler provides a better quality spectral velocity tracing but continuous wave (CW) Doppler can pick up higher velocities. The following calculations are used :

RV pressure – RA pressure

= Pressure gradient (PG) across tricuspid valve.

RV pressure

= PG + RA pressure (RAP)

(PG = 4 V_{max}^2: Bernoulli equation)

= 4V $_{max}^2$ + RAP

= Pulmonary artery pressure

(if no pulmonary stenosis)

RAP is normally < 5 mm and equal to the jugular venous pressure (JVP) which is assessed clinically. RAP can also be calculated from the inferior vena cava diameter in expiration (Fig. 9.4) and percentage collapse of IVC in inspiration, as shown in Table 9.1.

Table 9.1: Estimating right atrial pressure from the inferior vena cava		
IVC diameter (expiration)	*% age collapse (inspiration)*	*Right atrial pressure(RAP)*
<2 cm	100	<5 mm
<2 cm	>50	5-10 mm
>2 cm	25-50	10-15 mm
>2 cm	<25	15-20 mm

If transtricuspid Vmax is > 2.5 m/sec with RAP of 5mm or more, the pulmonary artery pressure(PAP) is elevated, as per the following calculations:

$$PAP = 4 \times (2.5)^2 + RAP$$
$$= 4 \times 6.25 + RAP$$
$$= 25 + 5 = 30 \text{ mm}.$$

- The normal pulmonary artery systolic velocity profile on Doppler is symmetrical and bullet shaped. In the presence of pulmonary hypertension it is asymmetrical with rapid peaking and a short acceleration time (AT) (Fig. 9.5). A time to peak pulmonary artery velo-

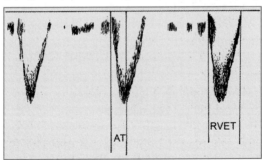

Fig. 9.5: Pulmonary artery velocity profile showing rapid peaking due to short acceleration time in a patient with pulmonary hypertension

city < 80 msec is indicative of pulmonary hypertension.

Causes of Pulmonary Hypertension

- Increased pulmonary flow
  Lt. to Rt. shunt: ASD, VSD, PDA.
- Raised left atrial pressure
  Mitral valve disease, LV dysfunction.
- Chronic pulmonary disease
  Bronchitis, Emphysema, Fibrosis.
- Obstruction to pulmonary flow
  thromboembolic, veno-occlusive disease
- Primary pulmonary hypertension.

Differential Diagnosis of Pulmonary Hypertension

- Pulmonary hypertension is a cause of right ventricular pressure overload. This is characterized by RV dilatation with or without RV hypertrophy and paradoxical IVS motion. A similar picture is observed in pulmonary stenosis with the difference that there is thickening and doming of pulmonary leaflets and the 'a' wave is prominent. (see Valvular Diseases)
- Pulmonary hypertension also needs to be differentiated from right ventricular volume overload. This is characterized by RV dilatation, minimal RV hypertrophy and paradoxical IVS motion. The situation is similar to differentiation between effect of systemic hypertension on the left ventricle from that of mitral regurgitation (see Systemic Hypertension). Because of technical difficulties in visualizing the right ventricle,

this differentiation requires expertise. Causes of RV volume overload are:

from right atrium	atrial septal defect (ASD) and tricuspid regurgitation (TR)
from left ventricle	ventricular septal defect (VSD)
from pulm. artery	pulmonary regurgitation (PR)
from aortic root	rupture sinus of Valsalva.

- A combination of a left-to-right shunt with pulmonary hypertension is referred to as Eisenmenger reaction. The level of shunt may be an atrial septal defect (ASD), a ventricular septal defect (VSD) or a patent ductus arteriosus (PDA). These conditions can be diagnosed by their specific echo features (see Congenital Heart Diseases).

- Besides pulmonary stenosis and RV volume over-load, pulmonary hypertension needs to be differen-tiated from other causes of paradoxical IVS motion such as:

    constrictive pericarditis
    after cardiac surgery
    left bundle branch block
    old septal infarction.

- Dilatation of the pulmonary artery observed in pulmo-nary hypertension is also seen in other conditions such as:

    pulmonary stenosis (post-stenotic dilatation)
    RV volume overload -VSD, ASD, TR.
    idiopathic dilatation of pulmonary artery.

CHAPTER TEN

AORTIC DISEASES

Normal Dimensions (Fig. 10.1)

Aortic annulus	17-25 mm
Sinus of Valsalva	22-36 mm
Sinotubular junction	18-26 mm
Aortic root width	20-37 mm
Anterior aortic swing	7-15 mm

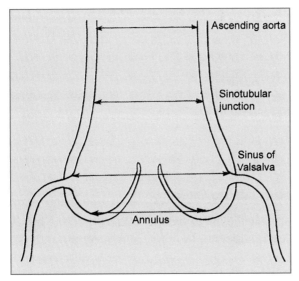

Fig. 10.1: Dimensions of the proximal aorta

Diameter of Aortic Annulus

The aortic annulus diameter is measured for the following purposes:

- to calculate the cardiac output from the cross-sectional area of the aortic valve (see Ventricular Dysfunction)

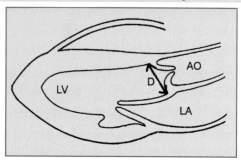

Fig. 10.2: Measurement of aortic annulus diameter from the PLAX view

- to determine the aortic valve area in aortic stenosis and to quantify aortic regurgitation from the width of the Doppler jet (see Valvular Diseases).
- to select the correct size of a prosthetic valve at the aortic position (Fig. 10.2).

Anterior Aortic Swing

- Normally the aorta swings anteriorly during left atrial filling in diastole, by 7 to 15 mm. An anterior aortic swing < 7 mm indicates a low cardiac ouput state and when > 15 mm it is a marker of hyperdynamic circulation.

Dilatation of Sinus of Valsalva

- Dilatation of the sinus of Valsalva beyond 40 mm is abnormal. An aneurysm of sinus of Valsalva appears as an outpouching of the dilated coronary sinus anterior to the anterior aortic wall protruding into the right ventricular outflow tract (RVOT) (Fig. 10.3). A

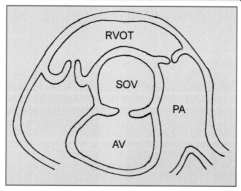

Fig. 10.3: Aneurysm of sinus of Valsalva (SOV) anterior to aortic valve (AV) protruding into the RV outflow tract

rupture of this aneurysm into the right ventricle produces right ventricular volume overload. Aneurysm of sinus of Valsalva or the fistula created by its rupture is best visualized on transoesophageal echo.

- Abnormalities associated with aneurysm of sinus of Valsalva include:

  Bicuspid aortic valve

  Coarctation of aorta

  Ventricular septal defect.

Aortic Atheromatous Plaque

- An aortic atheroma in the ascending or descending aorta appears as a mass protruding into the lumen on a cross-sectional view of the aorta. Transoesophageal echo is required to visualize the descending thoracic aorta. Echo can identify atheromatous plaques that are likely to cause peripheral embolization. In general, plaques that are large (> 5 mm in depth), mobile, pedunculated and with an ulcerated surface have a higher likelihood to embolize.

Dilatation of Aortic Root

- The normal diameter of the aortic root in end-diastole, between the leading edges of anterior and posterior aortic walls is 20 to 37 mm. Dilatation beyond 40 mm but less than 60 mm (Fig. 10.4) is observed in the following conditions:

Atherosclerosis	Aortic unfolding (old age) hypertension (ISH)
Medial necrosis	Marfan's syndrome Ehlers-Danlos syndrome
Aortitis	Syphilitic (rare) Tubercular Takayasu's disease
Collagenosis	Reiter's syndrome Ankylosing spondylitis.
Post-stenotic	Aortic stenosis.

- In aortic dilatation due to old age or hypertension, the aortic annulus and sinus of Valsalva are normal

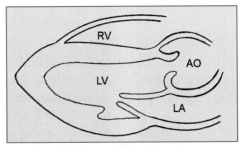

Fig. 10.4: PLAX view showing dilatation of the aortic root in a case of long-standing hypertension

in diameter. In medial necrosis, aortitis and collagen diseases, they are dilated and associated with aortic regurgitation. In post-stenotic aortic dilatation, there are features of valvular stenosis.

Aortic Aneurysm

- Dilatation of the aortic root beyond 60 mm is observed in aneurysmal dilatation of the aorta which may be saccular on fusiform (Fig. 10.5). The dilated aorta compresses the left atrium and expands in systole. The aortic cusps appear distant from the aortic walls even when the valve is open in systole. There may be an associated laminated thrombus.
- Causes of aortic aneurysm are:
  Atherosclerosis
  Syphilitic aortitis
  Marfan's syndrome
  Post-traumatic and
  Mycotic aneurysm.

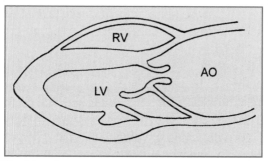

Fig. 10.5: PLAX view showing aneurysmal dilatation of the aorta in a case of Marfan's syndrome

Coarctation of Aorta

- In coarctation, there is a localized reduction of the aortic arch diameter with focal thickening and increased echo-reflectivity. The narrowing is at the juxta-ductal area (near the ductus arteriosus), proximal to the ligamentum arteriosum in pre-ductal coarctation and distal to it in post-ductal coarctation. There is post-stenotic dilatation of the descending aorta.
- The effects of aortic coarctation on the left ventricle are similar to those of systemic hypertension and aortic valve stenosis. There is left ventricular hypertrophy due to LV systolic (pressure) overload. There is thickening of the IV septum and LV posterior wall exceeding 12 mm with good LV systolic function. (see Systemic Hypertension).
- The narrowing of the aorta is detected from the suprasternal notch. The aortic arch is more pulsatile proximal to the coarctation than distal to it. On conti-nuous wave (CW) Doppler, there is a high velocity jet away from the transducer from which the pressure gradient across the coarctation can be determined (Fig. 10.6).
- Abnormalities associated with coarctation of aorta include:
  VSD and PDA
  Bicuspid aortic valve
  Aneurysm sinus of Valsalva
- In pseudo-coarctation of the aorta, there is only tucking at the ligamentum arteriosum without luminal

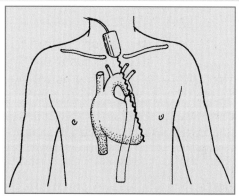

Fig. 10.6: Coarctation of aorta showing a high velocity jet on CW Doppler, with the transducer in the suprasternal notch

narrowing. In a condition known as hypoplastic aorta, there is diffuse narrowing of the aortic root lumen.

Aorto-septal Discontinuity

- Normally, the anterior wall of the aorta is continuous with the interventricular septum (IVS) on the parasternal long-axis (PLAX) view. The aorta overrides the IVS due to rightward displacement in Fallot's tetralogy. Discontinuity between the aorta and the IVS brings the aortic valve closure point in line with the IVS.
- Aorto-septal discontinuity is also observed with a subaortic type of ventricular septal defect (VSD).

Aortic Dissection

- Dissection of aorta is caused by cleavage of the media of the aortic wall with the adventitia and outer media forming the outer wall and the intima and inner

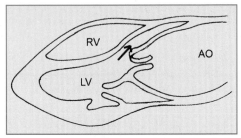

Fig. 10.7: Dissection of aorta forming a false lumen in the anterior aortic wall. An intimal flap separates the true and false lumens

media forming the inner wall. A false lumen appears between the two walls which has one blind end while the other end communicates with the true lumen at the site of the tear. The intimal flap oscillates between the true and false lumens (Fig. 10.7).

- Classical echo features of aortic dissection are:
  Dilatation of aortic root   > 42 mm
  Anterior or posterior wall thickness > 15 mm
  Double echo of the aortic wall with > 5 mm
  Separation between outer and inner walls.
  False lumen within aortic wall with blind end.
  Intimal flap between true and false lumens.
- Associated echo features of aortic dissection are:
  Occlusion of head and neck vessels
  Aortic valve regurgitation
  Left ventricular dysfunction
  Myocardial infarction
  Pericardial effusion
- Transoesophageal echo is the best technique for the diagnosis of aortic dissection. Dissection of the descending thoracic aorta can only be identified by this method.

De Bakey type	Stanford group	Location	Incidence
I ⎤	A	Ascending to descending aorta	10%
II ⎦		Confined to ascending aorta	70%
III	B	Confined to descending aorta	20%

Classification of aortic dissection

Causes of Aortic Dissection

- Marfan's syndrome
- Coarctation of aorta
- Hypertension in pregnancy
- Trauma: accidental/surgical.

Echo Features of Marfan's Syndrome

- Aortic root dilatation
- Aneurysm ascending aorta
- Aortic dissection
- Aortic regurgitation
- Mitral/tricuspid prolapse.

CHAPTER ELEVEN

CONGENITAL HEART DISEASES

Echo is a first-line and indispensible investigation for the diagnosis of congenital heart diseases. Not only can it localize an anatomical abnormality, it can also provide information about the effects of the abnormality on various cardiac chambers and can quantify intra-cardiac pressures such as the pulmonary artery pressure. In fact echocardiography has obviated the frequent need for cardiac catheterization, especially since some congenital defects are amenable to percutaneous catheter-guided closures. Examples of these are closure of an atrial septal defect and patent ductus arteriosus.

A detailed description of complex congenital cardiac abnormalities such as transposition of great vessels, is beyond the scope of this book. We shall confine our-selves to a discussion on the following congenital heart diseases:

   I. Ventricular septal defect   (VSD)
   II. Atrial septal defect   (ASD)
   III. Patent ductus arteriosus   (PDA)
   IV. Tetralogy of Fallot   (TOF)

Certain other congenital cardiac abnormalities find mention in other chapters of this book.

These are:

1. Coarctation of aorta (see Aortic Diseases)
2. Bicuspid aortic valve
3. Pulmonary stenosis
4. Ebstein's anomaly (see Valvular Diseases)

VENTRICULAR SEPTAL DEFECT

In this condition, a breach in the continuity of the inter-ventricular septum (IVS) creates a communication between the left and right ventricles. Flow of blood from the left ventricle (higher pressure) to the right ventricle (lower pressure) constitutes a left-to-right shunt across the ventricular septal defect (VSD).

2-D Echo

- On 2-D Echo, the left-sided chambers (LA and LV) are dilated, due to increased venous return from the pulmonary circulation: left ventricular volume over-load.

- On careful inspection of the apical 4-chamber (AP4CH) view, there is an echo drop-out in the inter-ventricular septum. The VSD may be small or large in size and single or multiple. The septal defect may be in the upper membranous portion or in the lower muscular septum. Rarely, the VSD is sub-aortic or supracristal in location. No echo drop-out is observed in VSD if the defect is too small (<3 mm) in size or trabecular (muscular) in location which shuts off during muscular contraction in systole.

Doppler Echo

- On colour flow mapping, there is an abnormal flow pattern from the left to right ventricle (Fig. 11.1). The width of the colour flow map approximates the size of the defect and helps in the quantitative assessment of the VSD.

- On continuous wave (CW) Doppler, a high velocity jet is identified across the defect. From the velocity (V) of the jet, the pressure gradient (PG) between the LV and RV can be measured (Bernoulli equation: $PG = 4\ V^2$). High velocity jet with a high pressure

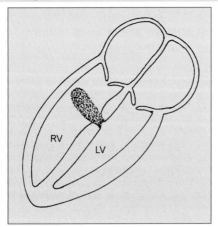

Fig. 11.1: Continuous wave (CW) Doppler showing high velocity flow across a ventricular septal defect from left to right ventricle

gradient is suggestive of a small restrictive VSD in the muscular portion of the septum. A shunt may not be demonstrated if it is small, of low velocity or bidirectional.

- By pulsed wave (PW) Doppler, the velocity picked up on CW Doppler and the abnormal signal obtained by colour flow mapping, can be localized. In this way, the site of the VSD is accurately identified.
- With a significant left-to-right shunt, there are features of right ventricular volume overload which include right ventricular dilatation >23 mm and paradoxical motion of the IV septum.

Doppler Calculations

- The pulmonary artery pressure can be estimated from the transtricuspid peak flow velocity and pulmonary hypertension can be identified (see Pulmonary Hypertension). A combination of VSD with pulmonary hypertension is known as Eisenmenger reaction (see below).

- The quantity of left-to-right shunt can be estimated from the ratio of pulmonary-to-systemic stroke volume, that is the Qp: Qs ratio (see below). Qs is aortic outflow and Qp is pulmonary outflow. Qp is greater than Qs since part of the left ventricular output goes to the right ventricle.

ATRIAL SEPTAL DEFECT

In this condition a breach in the continuity of the inter-atrial septum (IAS) creates a communication between the left and right atria. Flow of blood from the left atrium (higher pressure) to the right atrium (lower pressure) constitutes a left-to-right shunt across the atrial septal defect (ASD).

2-D Echo

- On 2-D echo, the right-sided chambers (RA and RV) are dilated due to increased venous return from the systemic circulation as well as the left atrium: right ventricular volume overload (Fig. 11.2).

- On careful inspection of the apical 4-chamber view, there is an echo drop-out in the interatrial septum. Since the IAS is thin and not perpendicular to the scanning beam, the reflected echo signal from the IAS is weak. Therefore, false echo drop-out may be observed even in normal individuals in the region of the foramen ovale. The subcostal view is better for

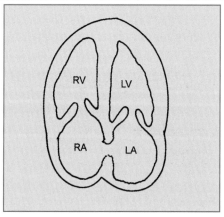

Fig. 11.2: Apical 4-chamber (AP4CH) view showing dilatation of right atrium and right ventricle with a defect in the interatrial septum

examining the IAS since it is perpendicular to the scanning beam. Transoesophageal echo allows excellent visualization of the IAS and thus a more accurate diagnosis of ASD and patent foramen ovale (PFO).

- The echo drop-out is seen in the middle of the IAS in ostium secondum type of ASD and just above the mitral valve ring in ostium primum type of ASD. No echo drop-out is observed in the sinus venosus type of ASD and in anomalous pulmonary venous drainage (APVD). In them, other features of a left-to-right shunt are nevertheless present.
- With a significant left-to-right shunt, there are features of right ventricular volume overload which include right ventricular dilatation >23 mm and paradoxical motion of the IV septum.

Doppler Echo

- Doppler study is not a good modality to pick up an ASD because the jet across the defect is of low velocity. For the same reason, colour flow mapping can detect flow from the left to right atrium in only a minority of ASDs.
- In ostium primum type of ASD, there may be associated mitral and tricuspid regurgitation (MR and TR) due to cleft valve leaflets.

Contrast Echo

- Because of the technical difficulties with 2-D Echo and the limitations of colour flow mapping and Doppler echo, a contrast echo study should be performed if an ASD is strongly suspected. For contrast study, a small bolus of agitated saline having air bubbles, is injected into a peripheral vein. The air bubbles are seen in the right atrium (RA) and then they enter the right ventricle. The subject is asked to perform a Valsalva manoeuvre (to increase intrathoracic pressure) when air bubbles are seen shunting from the right to left atrium. This is known as a positive contrast effect. A negative contrast effect is observed when there is an area of non-contrast in the RA due to washout of contrast by normal blood from the LA.

Doppler Calculations

- The pulmonary artery pressure can be estimated from the transtricuspid peak flow velocity and pulmonary hypertension can be identified (see

Pulmonary Hypertension). A combination of ASD with pulmonary hypertension is known as Eisenmenger reaction (see below).

- The quantity of left-to-right shunt can be estimated from the ratio of pulmonary-to-systemic stroke volume, that is the Qp: Qs ratio (see below). Qs is aortic outflow and Qp is pulmonary outflow. Qp is greater than Qs since part of the left atrial output goes to the right atrium.

PATENT DUCTUS ARTERIOSUS

In this condition, the ductus arteriosus fails to close after birth and thus provides a communication between the aorta and the pulmonary artery. Flow of blood from the aorta (higher pressure) to the pulmonary artery (lower pressure) constitutes a left-to-right shunt across the patent ductus arteriosus (PDA).

2-D Echo

- On 2-D echo, the left-sided chambers (LA and LV) are dilated due to increased venous return from the pulmonary circulation: left ventricular volume over-load.
- Due to dilatation of the left atrium, the ratio between left atrial and aortic diameters (LA : AO ratio) exceeds 1.15.

Doppler Echo

- On colour flow mapping using the parasternal short-axis (PSAX) view, there is a jet in the pulmonary artery with a prominent diastolic flow (Fig. 11.3). It

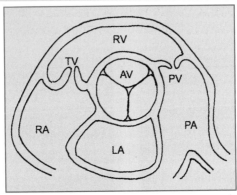

Fig. 11.3: Parasternal short-axis (PSAX) view at the aortic valve (AV) level showing the pulmonary artery and its branches

can be differentiated from the adjacent jet of pulmonary regurgitation (PR) by the fact that in PDA, there is no flow in the right ventricular outflow tract (RVOT).

Doppler Calculations

- The pulmonary artery pressure can be estimated from the transtricuspid peak flow velocity and pulmonary hypertension can be identified (see Pulmonary Hypertension). A combination of PDA with pulmonary hypertension is known as Eisenmenger reaction (see below).
- The quantity of left-to-right shunt can be estimated from the ratio of pulmonary-to-systemic stroke volume, that is the Qp: Qs ratio (see below). Qs is pulmonary outflow or tricuspid inflow before receiving blood from the aorta through the ductus. Qp is mitral inflow or aortic outflow after receiving blood from the

aorta. Qp is greater than Qs since part of the aortic blood goes to the pulmonary artery.

TETRALOGY OF FALLOT

Although discussion of complex congenital cardiac abnormalities is beyond the scope of this book, one condition that deserves mention is tetralogy of Fallot (Fig. 11.4). The four components of the tetralogy are:

1. *Ventricular septal defect (VSD)*
   The VSD is usually membranous in location.
2. *Overriding aorta (OA)*
   There is rightward displacement of the aorta and discontinuity between the aorta and the IV septum

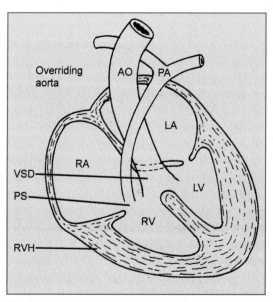

Fig. 11.4: The four components of Fallot's tetralogy

(aorta-septal discontinuity). The IV septum is thus in line with the aortic valve closure point and not the anterior aortic wall.

3. *Right ventricular outflow tract obstruction (RVOTO)*

   RVOT obstruction is often infundibular (subvalvular) in location and uncommonly due to valvular pulmonary stenosis.

4. *Right ventricular hypertrophy (RVH)*

   The right ventricular chamber undergoes hypertrophy in response to pulmonary stenosis. The RV free wall thickness is > 5 mm and there is paradoxical motion of the IV septum. Importantly, the left-sided chambers (LA and LV) are normal or smaller in size in contrast to their larger size in some other left-to-right shunts.

EISENMENGER REACTION

- When there is a shunt between cardiac chambers or blood vessels, blood will flow from a region of higher pressure (left side) to a region of lower pressure (right side). This constitutes a left-to-right shunt. When there is significant quantity of shunting, it leads to right ventricular volume overload and RV dilatation. Further, when irreversible changes occur in the pulmonary vasculature, pulmonary vascular resistance rises and pulmonary arterial hypertension occurs. A combination of a shunt with pulmonary hypertension is referred to as Eisenmenger reaction. Ultimately, when right-sided pressures exceed left-sided pressures, reversal of shunt occurs. This constitutes a right-to-left shunt.

- In the presence of a cardiac shunt, the pulmonary artery pressure can be estimated from the trans-tricuspid peak flow velocity (Vmax).

- Features of right ventricular volume overload include right ventricular dilatation >23 mm and paradoxical motion of the IV septum.
- When reversal of shunt occurs, colour flow mapping shows a bidirectional shunt or a low velocity jet from the right to left side of the defect.

QUANTIFICATION OF SHUNT

- The stroke volume of the left heart and thus the cardiac output (cardiac output = stroke volume × heart rate) can be calculated from the peak aortic flow velocity. This is obtained by Doppler spectral display of aortic outflow tract in the apical 5-chamber view. The area under curve of this velocity display is the flow velocity integral (FVI). Multiplying this FVI with the cross-sectional area (CSA) of the aortic valve yields the stroke volume (SV). Cross-sectional area (CSA) is obtained from the diameter (D) of the aortic annulus.

    $SV = CSA \times FVI$
    $= 0.785 \, D^2 \times FVI$
    (See Ventricular Dysfunction).

- Using similar calculations on the peak pulmonary flow velocity, the stroke volume of the right heart can be obtained. If the quantum of systemic flow is Qs and the quantum of pulmonary flow is Qp, the Qp: Qs ratio is a measure of the quantity of shunt. A shunt is haemodynamically significant if the shunt ratio (Qp: Qs) exceeds 2.0.

$$\frac{Qp}{Qs} = \frac{FVIp \times D^2 p}{FVIs \times D^2 s}$$

- In VSD, Qs is AV flow and Qp is PV or MV flow. Part of left ventricular output is lost to the right ventricle. Pulmonary outflow and mitral inflow are the same.
- In ASD Qs is AV flow and Qp is PV or TV flow. Part of left atrial output is lost to the right atrium. Pulmonary outflow and tricuspid inflow are the same.
- In PDA Qs is PV or TV flow before receiving blood from the ductus and Qp is MV or AV flow after receiving blood from the ductus. TV inflow and PV outflow are the same. MV inflow and AV outflow are the same.

CHAPTER TWELVE

VALVULAR DISEASES

One of the earliest applications of echocardiography was in the diagnosis of valvular diseases in general and mitral stenosis in particular. In fact even today, after coronary artery disease and systemic hypertension, suspected disease of cardiac valves is a common indication for requesting an echo. Often valvular disease is suspected clinically because of a murmur especially if coupled with suggestive symptoms such as dyspnoea and palpitation on exertion. A murmur is a sound caused by turbulent blood flow due to:

high volume flow across a normal valve

high velocity flow across a stenotic valve

regurgitant flow from an incompetent valve

Sometimes a murmur is caused by an intracardiac left-to-right shunt or a narrowed major blood vessel (see Congenital Heart Diseases).

Echocardiography can confirm the site of origin of a murmur detected clinically. It can image a diseased valve and detect an abnormal pattern of blood flow on colour flow mapping. It can also reveal the etiology of the valvular disease, quantify its severity and assess its effect on dimensions of cardiac chambers and on ventricular function.

MITRAL STENOSIS

Echo Features of MS

2-D Echo PLAX View

• The mitral valve leaflets are thickened due to dense fibrosis, with or without calcification. Due to fibrosis, their echogenicity (brightness) is increased and equals that of the pericardium. When there is

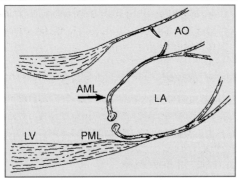

Fig. 12.1: Illustration of the mitral valve in mitral stenosis showing:
A. Thickening of the valve leaflets,
B. Diastolic doming of anterior leaflet,
C. Restricted opening of the valve,
D. dilatation of the left atrium

associated calcification, echogenicity exceeds that of the pericardium and there is distal shadowing. Instead of a sharp image of leaflets, there is reverberation of echoes with several reflections giving a fuzzy image.

- There is limited excursion of mitral leaflets with restricted valve opening. Due to fusion at the free edges and anterior motion of the body of anterior mitral leaflet (AML), there is diastolic doming of AML (Fig. 12.1). This is described as a "bent-knee motion" or "elbowing" of AML and is likened to the bulging of a boat's sail as it fills with wind.

- There is dilatation of the left atrium (normal size 19-40 mm). There may be a left atrial thrombus especially in the presence of atrial fibrillation. Other causes of LA dilatation are mitral regurgitation (MR) and LV dysfunction.

- There may be thickening and increased echogenicity of the chordae tendinae if there is an associated significant subvalvular disease.

M-mode AV Level

- There is dilatation of the left atrium (normal LA size: 19-40 mm). There may be a left atrial thrombus.
- There may be thickening of aortic valve leaflets due to associated aortic stenosis.

M-mode MV Level

- The D-E excursion of the anterior mitral leaflet (AML) is reduced to less than 20 mm (normal 20-35 mm). Reduced AML DE excursion is also seen in low cardiac output states.
- There is loss of the normal antiparallel motion of the posterior mitral leaflet (PML) in diastole. This is known as paradoxical anterior motion of PML which is pulled towards the AML rather than drifting away from it. It occurs because of fusion between the edges of AML and PML with the PML following the larger and more mobile AML.
- There is flattening of the E-F slope (normal 80-120 mm/sec) due to slow and continued left ventricular filling during diastole. Flattening of E-F slope is also seen with reduced left ventricular compliance (Fig. 12.2).

M-mode LV Level

- In pure mitral stenosis, left ventricular dimensions and function are normal. If there is associated mitral

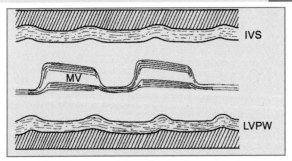

Fig. 12.2: M-mode scan at the mitral valve level showing:
    A. Reverberation of echoes from the valve,
    B. Reduced anterior excursion of the AML,
    C. Paradoxical anterior motion of the PML,
    D. Flattening of the E-F slope of AML

regurgitation, there are features of left ventricular volume overload.

- When mitral stenosis leads to pulmonary hypertension, there is dilatation of the right ventricle (more than 23 mm) and paradoxical motion of the interventricular septum (see Pulmonary Hypertension).

2-D Echo PSAX View

- At the aortic valve level, there may be thickening of the cusps due to associated aortic valve stenosis. The enlarged left atrium is visualized along with its appendage in this view. There may be a thrombus in the left atrium or in its appendage.

- At the mitral valve level, there is thickening and reduced excursion of mitral leaflets. The normal 'fish-mouth like' opening of the mitral valve orifice is restricted (Fig. 12.3). At this level, the mitral valve area can be measured by planimetry (tracing of the

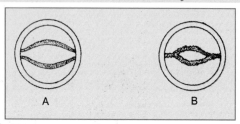

Fig. 12.3: Illustration of the mitral valve on
short-axis view showing:
A. Normal "fish-mouth like" opening,
B. Reduced mitral valve orifice size

valve orifice area). The normal mitral orifice area is
4-6 cm² or 3 cm² per square metre body surface area
(BSA).

Colour Flow Mapping

- On the AP4CH view, there is a "candle-flame like" jet
  with aliasing in the centre, at the plane of the mitral
  valve (Fig. 12.4). The jets extend lower down beyond

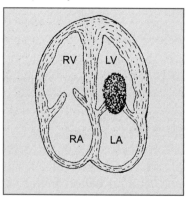

Fig. 12.4: Colour flow mapping from the apical 4-chamber
view showing a jet in the mitral valve

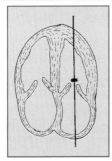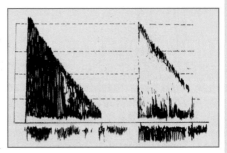

Fig. 12.5: Pulsed-wave (PW) Doppler from the apical 4-chamber view showing increased diastolic flow velocity across the mitral valve with slow deceleration

the MV plane and is often eccentric if there is significant subvalvular disease.

- The width of the colour flow jet approximates the diameter of the valve and gives an idea about the severity of MS.

Doppler Echo

- On PW Doppler from the AP4CH view with the sample volume in LV, the MV inflow spectral trace shows an increased peak diastolic flow velocity exceeding 1 m/sec (normal velocity: 0.6-1.4 m/sec; mean 0.9 m/sec). There is a slow decay of the velocity with a flat slope of deceleration (Fig. 12.5). The mean pressure gradient across the valve exceeds 4 mmHg.

Doppler Calculations

- Because of the stenosed valve, the time taken for the pressure gradient across the valve to fall, is

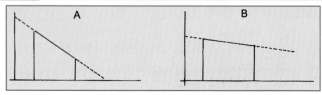

Fig. 12.6: Relationship between rate of velocity deceleration and severity of mitral stenosis:
A. steep slope: mild MS,
B. flat slope: severe MS

prolonged. Greater the degree of stenosis, more is the prolongation (Fig. 12.6). This fact is utilized to estimate the mitral valve area from the pressure half-time. The pressure half-time is the time taken for the peak pressure gradient to fall by half. Because of the square relationship between pressure and velocity (Bernaulli Equation: $P = 4V^2$), the pressure half-time is the time for peak velocity to fall to 0.7 of its original value (Fig. 12.7).

$P \alpha V^2$ therefore $1/2\ P \alpha V^2/2 \alpha V/\sqrt{2}$

$\alpha V/1.4 \alpha V \times 0.7$

MV area (cm^2) = 220/P 1/2 t (millisec)

220 is the Hatle's constant

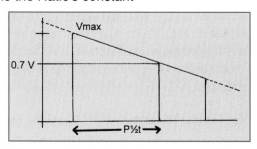

Fig. 12.7: The principle of calculating pressure half-time (P½t)

Note:

1. This formula should not be applied in mild mitral stenosis (P 1/2 t < 150 millisec) since the P 1/2 t is then related to the diastolic behaviour of the left atrium and left ventricle.

2. In the presence of atrial fibrillation, when the duration of diastole varies from beat-to-beat, a number of beats should be used for calculation and the average value of MV area should be taken.

- The pulmonary artery pressure can be estimated from the transtricuspid flow velocity (Vmax) obtained from the Doppler spectral display added to the right atrial pressure. A Vmax more than 2.5 m/sec is suggestive of pulmonary hypertension (see Pulmonary Hypertension).

Pitfalls in the Diagnosis of MS

- Some of the echo features of mitral stenosis are not specific for this condition. Limited excursion of mitral valve leaflets with restricted valve opening is also observed in low cardiac output states.
- Diastolic doming of the AML is also due to redundant leaflet tissue in mitral valve prolapse and vegetations on the free edge of AML in endocarditis. Reduced D-E excursion is also due to low cardiac output and flattening of E-F slope is also due to reduced left ventricular compliance.
- For measurement of mitral valve area by planimetry, the short axis cut must be taken at the level of leaflet edges, which is the smallest area. Taking the cut at

the level of leaflet doming may falsely suggest a larger area. It may be difficult to trace the orifice accurately if the lumen is irregular and there are reverberation artefacts due to heavy calcification. In that case, the severity of mitral stenosis is likely to be overestimated.

- The transmitral peak velocity and pressure gradient depend upon the heart rate and stroke volume. These are overestimated in the presence of tachycardia (shorter diastole) and a high output state (greater blood flow). Conversely, the velocity and pressure gradient are reduced in the presence of bradycardia and a low output state.

Severity of MS

- The severity of MS as per mitral valve area (MVA), pressure half-time (P ½t) and transtricuspid velocity (TR Vmax) can be graded as shown in Table 12.1.

Table 12.1: MS severity from pressure half-time and transtricuspid velocity			
Severity of MS	*MVA (cm²)*	*P ½t (msec)*	*TR Vmax (m/sec)*
Mild MS	1.5-2.5	< 150	< 2.7
Moderate MS	1.0-1.5	150-220	2.7-3.0
Severe MS	< 1.0	> 220	> 3.0

Criteria for Severe MS

MV orifice area	<1 cm²
Mean pressure gradient	>10 mmHg
Pressure half-time	> 220 msec

Tricuspid flow velocity   > 3 m/sec
Pulmonary artery pressure   > 30 mmHg

Causes of MS

Practically speaking, the commonest cause of MS is rheumatic heart disease.

Much rarer causes of MS are:

    Mitral annulus calcification (in the elderly)
    Congenital mitral stenosis (parachute valve)
    Connective tissue disorders (SLE, rheumatoid)
    Mucopolysaccharidosis (Hurler's syndrome)

Other rarer causes of mitral inflow obstruction are:

    Left atrial myxoma
    Left atrial thrombus
    Cor-triatriatum
    Supravalvular ring.

Suitability for Valvotomy in MS

Often conventional echocardiography is performed in a known case of mitral stenosis, to assess whether the valve is suitable for balloon valvotomy. This is a specialized judgement that often requires subsequent trans-oesophageal echocardiography (TOE). In general, a valve is suitable for balloon valvotomy if there is significant mitral stenosis but without the following:

• immobility of leaflet base
• thickening of the chordae
• commissural calcification
• more than mild MR
• left atrial thrombus.

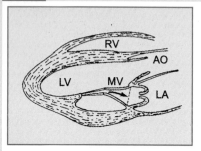

Fig. 12.8: Parasternal long-axis view showing systolic bowing of both mitral leaflets, above the annular plane and into the left atrium

MITRAL VALVE PROLAPSE

Echo Features of MVP

2-D Echo PLAX View

- The mitral valve leaflets are thick and redundant (due to myxomatous degeneration) with increased echogenicity.
- There is a systolic bowing movement of part of either or both leaflets above the plane of the mitral valve annulus (Fig. 12.8). According to the extent of motion, mitral valve prolapse can be classified into the following types:

  Type 1: AML and PML move up to annulus in late systole

  Type 2: Large AML bows into left atrium overshooting PML

  Type 3: AML and PML both prolapse into the left atrium.

M-Mode MV Level

- There is an abrupt posterior displacement of one or both leaflets in systole. In Type 2 MVP, there is a late-systolic posterior bulge while in Type 3 MVP, there is

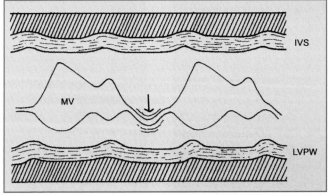

Fig. 12.9: M-mode scan at the mitral valve level showing hammock-like posterior motion of both leaflets in systole

a generalized hammock-like posterior motion throughout systole (Fig. 12.9).

- This is preceded by anterior buckling and exaggerated excursion of the large AML into the left ventricular outflow tract (LVOT). The increased excursion is because of redundancy of the leaflet.

2-D Echo-AP4CH View

- There is superior arching of the mitral valve leaflets into the left atrium.
- There may be an associated tricuspid valve prolapse in Marfan's syndrome.

Doppler Echo

- There are features of mitral regurgitation. On colour flow mapping, the regurgitant jet is often eccentric and slow in onset (midsystolic).

Pitfalls in the Diagnosis of MVP

- Nodular thickening of leaflets due to myxomatous degeneration may be mistaken for vegetations seen in endocarditis (see Endocarditis).
- Pseudoprolapse of the mitral valve may be observed in pericardial effusion (see Pericardial Diseases)
- Anterior buckling of the AML into the LVOT resembles systolic anterior motion (SAM) of AML seen in hypertrophic obstructive cardiomyopathy: HOCM (see Cardiomyopathies).
- Minor 'technical mitral valve prolapse' may be observed in normal persons due to high transducer position with caudal angulation. Alternatively, a true mitral valve prolapse may be missed due to low transducer position with cranial angulation.
- Mitral valve prolapse needs to be differentiated from a flail mitral valve leaflet caused by a ruptured papillary muscle or chordae tendinae (see below).

Causes of MV Prolapse

- Idiopathic myxomatous degeneration
- Rheumatic heart disease
- Ostium secundum ASD
- Primary pulmonary hypertension
- Ehlers-Danlos syndrome.

FLAIL MITRAL LEAFLET

Echo Features of Flail MV Leaflet

2-D Echo PLAX View

- The flail leaflet exhibits a free and exaggerated whip-like motion (like a sail flapping in the wind). The leaflet

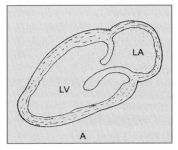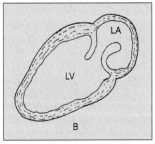

Fig. 12.10: A. Apical 2-chamber view showing a flail posterior mitral leaflet in the left ventricle,
B. that moves past the mitral annular plane into the left atrium

tip moves past the mitral annular plane, enters deep into the left atrium and fails to coapt with the other MV leaflet. The flail leaflet is generally the posterior mitral leaflet (PML) (Fig. 12.10).

M-mode MV Level

- There is a coarse diastolic flutter of the flail leaflet (Fig. 12.11). Erratic motion of the affected leaflet

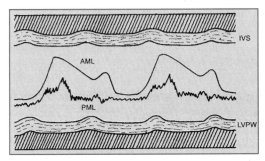

Fig. 12.11: M-mode scan at the mitral valve level showing coarse diastolic flutter of the flail posterior leaflet

causes a beat-to-beat variation of the MV diastolic pattern. The AML and PML separate at the onset of diastole and come together at the onset of systole.

- On M-mode scan at the AV level, fine lines with systolic vibration are seen in the left atrium, due to prolapse of the flail leaflet.

Doppler Echo

- On CW Doppler and colour flow mapping, there is a jet of mitral regurgitation. The MR jet is often eccentric and directed towards the posterior left atrial wall. The jet area may be less than that expected for the degree of MR. Therefore, there is a risk of underestimating the degree of mitral regurgitation.

Differential Diagnosis of Flail MV Leaflet

- A flail mitral valve leaflet needs to be differentiated from a prolapsed mitral valve leaflet. The differences between the two conditions are given in Table 12.2.

Table 12.2: Differences between flail mitral leaflet and prolapsed leaflet		
	Flail leaflet	*Prolapsed leaflet*
Range of motion	Flaps freely	Buckles/domes
Entry into left atrium		
extent	deep	just enters
duration	for long time	for short time
Direction of tip	towards LA	towards LV

- On M-mode scan at the MV level, multiple echoes of the flail PML may resemble those produced by a left atrial myxoma. The 2-D echo picture of these two conditions is, however, altogether different (see Intracardiac Masses).

Causes of Flail MV Leaflet

- Coronary artery disease: The commonest cause of a flail leaflet is rupture of a papillary muscle or chordae tendinae in a setting of acute myocardial infarction. Rupture of the posteromedial papillary muscle with a resultant flail PML generally follows inferior wall infarction. This causes acute mitral regurgitation (see Coronary Artery Disease)
- Other uncommon causes are:
  —bacterial endocarditis
  —connective tissue disorders
  —blunt chest-wall trauma.

MITRAL ANNULAR CALCIFICATION

Echo Features of MAC

2-D Echo PLAX View

- There is a localized highly reflective echodensity in the posterior segment of the mitral valve annulus. The calcification involves the base of the posterior mitral leaflet (PML) and extends into the left atrial wall and the basal portion of left ventricular posterior wall (LVPW). The architecture of the PML is distorted and it is rendered immobile (Fig. 12.12).
- There may be associated aortic annular calcification.

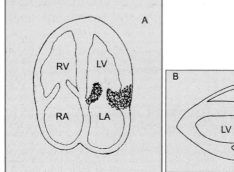

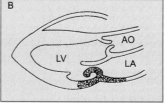

Fig. 12.12: Apical 4-chamber view:
A   Parasternal long-axis view
B   showing calcification of the mitral valve annulus

M-mode MV Level

- There is a thick dense band of echoes behind the mitral valve leaflets (AML and PML) reflected from the calcified mitral annulus.

Doppler Echo

- Mitral annular calcification may cause mild functional mitral regurgitation (MR). Rarely, it may lead to mild mitral stenosis (MS).

Pitfalls in the Diagnosis of MAC

- Calcified mitral annulus may be mistaken for the left ventricular posterior wall (LVPW). In that case, the LVPW may be misdiagnosed as a pericardial effusion (see Pericardial Diseases)
- Mistaking a calcified mitral annulus for the LVPW can cause error in the measurement of left ventricular

internal dimensions (LVESD and LVEDD) for assessment of left ventricular function (see Ventricular Dysfunction). The key feature of the LVPW as opposed to a calcified mitral annulus is that the LVPW thickens in systole.

- Ulcerated excrescences on a calcific mitral annulus may produce reverberation artefacts which resemble vegetations of endocarditis (see Endocarditis).

Cause of MAC

- Mitral annular calcification with mild mitral regurgitation is one of the commonest normal findings observed when echo is performed in elderly subjects.

MITRAL REGURGITATION

Echo Features of MR

M-mode LV Level

- The left ventricle is dilated and hyperkinetic due to volume overload (Fig. 12.13). This is to maintain

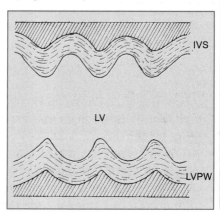

Fig. 12.13: M-mode scan at the ventricular level showing a dilated and hyperkinetic left ventricle with exaggerated excursion of its walls

cardiac output since a fraction of the stroke volume regurgitates into the left atrium. Similar overloading of the left ventricle is observed in aortic regurgitation.

- The amplitude of motion of the IV septum and LV posterior wall is exaggerated in MR due to valvular disease. In functional MR due to annular stretching, there may be global hypokinesia (cardiomyopathy) or regional wall motion abnormality (RWMA) due to old myocardial infarction.

2-D Echo PLAX View

- The left atrium (LA) is dilated (normal size 19-40 mm) with systolic expansion and increased LA posterior wall motion. Other causes of left atrial dilatation are mitral stenosis and LV dysfunction.
- The mitral valve architecture suggests the underlying cause of mitral regurgitation. There may be MV prolapse, flail MV leaflet, mitral annular calcification or vegetations on leaflets in endocarditis. Rheumatic MR is suggested by thickened and fibrosed leaflets.

M-mode MV Level

- Mitral valve leaflets show exaggerated excursion and quick MV closure due to rapid diastolic filling. Accordingly, the DE excursion of the AML is increased and the E-F slope is sharp (short deceleration time) (Fig. 12.14).
- There may be features of the underlying cause of MR such as MV prolapse or flail MV leaflet. MR of rheumatic aetiology is often associated with some degree of mitral stenosis (MS).

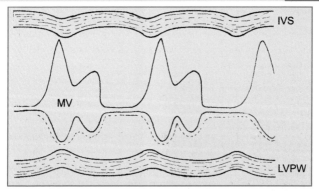

Fig. 12.14: M-mode scan at the mitral valve level showing exaggerated anterior motion (increased D-E excursion) and quick posterior motion (sleep E-F slope) of the anterior leaflet

M-mode LV Dimensions

- The left ventricular internal dimensions in end-diastole and end-systole (LVESD and LVEDD) are increased. Indices of left ventricular systolic function (FS and LVEF) suggesting good LV function. If mitral regurgitation is due to annular stretching (functional MR), LV systolic function is impaired (see Ventricular Function). There may be eccentric LV hypertrophy which is inadequate for the degree of LV dilatation, along with an increase in LV mass (see Systemic Hypertension).

M-mode AV Level

- Since a fraction of the stroke volume regurgitates into the left atrium, there is midsystolic closure of the aortic valve cusps. Other causes of midsystolic aortic valve closure are as follows:

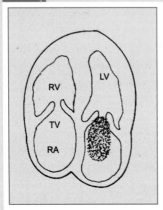

Fig. 12.15: Colour flow mapping from the apical 4-chamber view showing a MR jet in the left atrium

HOCM (dynamic LVOT obstruction)
AS (subvalvular aortic stenosis)
VSD (ventricular septal defect).

Colour Flow Mapping

• A regurgitant jet is seen in the left atrium on PLAX and AP4CH views (Fig. 12.15). The extent to which the MR jet fills the LA cavity indicates the severity of MR as shown in Table 12.3.

Table 12.3: Assessment of MR severity by colour flow mapping		
MR severity	*Area of colour (cm²)*	*% of LA area*
Mild	< 4	< 25
Moderate	4-8	25-50
Severe	> 8	> 50

• A turbulent jet with a swirling movement can cause systolic flow reversal in the pulmonary veins. This retrograde flow along with normal venous inflow sometimes gives a variance colour map.

- The width of the MR jet at the level of MV leaflet tips correlates with the degree of regurgitation. A broad colour flow signal (wide jet) represents severe MR.
- The spatial profile of the MR jet does not actually reflect the regurgitant volume. The profile of MR jet depends upon the following variables:
  — size and shape of the MV orifice
  — angle of jet in relation to MV
  — pressure difference across the MV
  — loading conditions and LV compliance
  — size and distensibility of left atrium.
- The MR jet is eccentric or off-centre in:
  — mitral valve prolapse
  — flail mitral leaflet
  — paraprosthetic leak.

Doppler Echo

- On CW Doppler, scanning the entire left atrium from the AP4CH view can detect the MR jet at any angle. The velocity of the MR jet exceeds 2 m/sec, but the severity of MR is not only related to the velocity. Rather, severity of MR is more closely related to the density or intensity of the flow signal. A dense or intense signal indicates that greater volume of blood is moving at a given velocity.
- By CW Doppler, the pulmonary artery pressure can be estimated from the transtricuspid flow velocity (Vmax) obtained from the spectral display added to the right atrial pressure. A Vmax more than

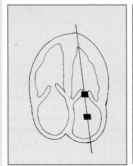 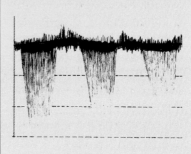

Fig. 12.16: Pulsed-wave (PW) Doppler from the apical 4-chamber view showing a MR flow signal in the left atrium

2.5 m/sec is suggestive of pulmonary hypertension (see Pulmonary Hypertension).

- On PW Doppler (Fig. 12.16), mapping progressively deeper into the left atrium (LA) till flow is not seen, can quantify the severity of MR as shown in Table 12.4.

Table 12.4: Assessment of MR severity by PW Doppler

MR severity	Depth of flow in LA
Mild	< 2 cm into LA
Moderate	> 2 cm up to mid-LA
Severe	Up to distal LA

- On PW Doppler, with the sample volume in a pulmonary vein, retrograde systolic flow (away from left atrium) may be detected.

Pitfalls in the Diagnosis of MR

- The spatial profile of the MR jet depends upon several variables and, therefore, does not truly reflect the actual regurgitant volume. The MR jet may be underestimated or even altogether missed if it is eccentric. This error can be avoided by scanning the entire left atrium, by placing the sample volume of PW Doppler in different locations.

- In acute MR due to papillary muscle rupture in a setting of acute MI, there is no time for LV and LA dilatation to develop. A small-volume high-velocity MR jet with normal MV architecture is observed causing an acute rise in left ventricular end-diastolic pressure (LVEDP) and pulmonary oedema.

- It may be difficult if not impossible to differentiate organic MR with LV dysfunction from a dilated cardio-myopathy (DCMP) with functional MR. Features in favour of organic MR are:
  — a long-standing pansystolic murmur
  — MV leaflet prolapse, flaility or thickening.

- In presence of MR, LV ejection fraction (LVEF) may be normal despite reduced LV contractility because the left atrium offers far less resistance to ejection than does the aorta. After mitral valve repair or replacement, the LVEF is likely to fall.

Criteria for Severe MR

- Colour flow jet filling 50% of left atrium
- Systolic flow reversal in pulmonary veins
- Dense flow signal on CW Doppler
- Flow up to distal LA on PW Doppler
- Left ventricular volume overload
- Raised pulmonary artery pressure.

Causes of MR

1. Rheumatic heart disease (with MS)
2. Mitral valve prolapse
3. Coronary artery disease:
   a. ischemic cardiomyopathy
   b. papillary muscle dysfunction
4. Mitral annular calcification
5. Cardiomyopathy:
   a. dilated CMP
   b. restrictive CMP
   c. hypertrophic CMP
6. Connective tissue disorders e.g.
   SLE, Marfan's Syndrome

Acute MR is caused by rupture of a papillary muscle or chordae tendinae leading to a flail mitral valve leaflet. Causes of acute MR are:

acute myocardial infarction
subacute bacterial endocarditis
blunt chest wall trauma.

TRICUSPID STENOSIS

Echo Features of TS

M-Mode and 2-D Echo

The 2-D and M-mode features of tricuspid stenosis are similar to those of mitral stenosis. These include:

- Thickened leaflets (due to fibrosis) with or without calcification, causing multiple reverberation echoes
- Limited excursion of leaflets with restricted valve opening and slow diastolic closure rate (flat EF slope) (Fig. 12.17).

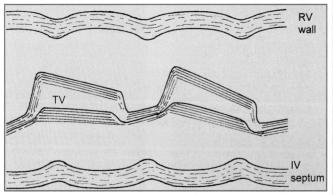

Fig. 12.17: M-mode scan of the tricuspid valve showing:
A. Multiple reverberation echoes,
B. limited leaflet excursion

- Diastolic doming of anterior tricuspid leaflet with paradoxical anterior motion of the septal tricuspid leaflet.

Unlike in mitral stenosis, the stenotic tricuspid orifice cannot be imaged. The tricuspid leaflets can be visualized in the apical 4-chamber view and in the parasternal short-axis view (aortic valve level) if the right ventricle is enlarged or if there is rotation of the heart due to emphysema and cor pulmonale. They are also visualized by M-mode scanning from the PLAX view, in the right ventricle anterior to the interventricular septum (IVS).

Doppler Echo

On PW Doppler, in the AP4CH view with the sample volume in the RV, the TV inflow spectral trace shows an increased peak diastolic flow velocity exceeding

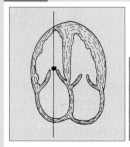 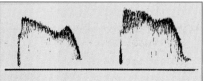

Fig. 12.18: Pulsed-wave (PW) Doppler from the apical 4-chamber view showing increased diastolic flow velocity across the tricuspid valve

0.5 m/sec (normal velocity: 0.3-0.7 m/sec) (Fig. 12.18). Evaluation of the severity of TS is rarely required clinically.

Causes of TS

- The commonest cause of TS is rheumatic heart disease. Almost always mitral stenosis coexists. MS is 10 times more common than TS.
  Other rare causes of tricuspid obstruction are:
  — carcinoid syndrome (with associated TR)
  — right atrial myxoma obstructing the TV
  — TV vegetation obstructing RV inflow tract
  — constrictive pericarditis involving A-V groove.

Clinical Significance of TS

- Rheumatic heart disease affects the right side of the heart much less commonly than it does the mitral and aortic valves.
- Tricuspid stenosis (TS) is difficult to diagnose clinically especially in the presence of mitral stenosis (MS).

- It is important to establish if the tricuspid valve is involved in rheumatic heart diseases, since even a small pressure gradient is haemodynamically significant.
- Echo can tell the diagnosis of TS but cannot assess its severity, since the stenotic tricuspid orifice cannot be visualized.

TRICUSPID REGURGITATION

Echo Features of TR

2-D Echo AP4CH View

- The right ventricle is dilated and hyperkinetic due to volume overload. It is of the same size or larger than the left ventricle. When enlarged, the right ventricle becomes globular and loses its normal triangular shape.
- The right atrium is dilated and shows systolic expansion with bulging of the interatrial septum towards the left atrium.

2-D Echo SC4CH View

- The dilated right ventricle and right atrium can also be visualized from the subcostal 4 chamber view (SC4CH view).
- Additionally, the inferior vena cava and hepatic veins are dilated with further expansion in systole due to regurgitation. The liver is pulsatile.

  Note: Regurgitation into the inferior vena cava (IVC) is also observed in cardiac tamponade and right ventricular dysfunction but in diastole. In these conditions, the IVC is dilated beyond 2 cm and fails to constrict by at least 50 percent during inspiration.

- Injection of a contrast agent in an upper limb vein can demonstrate reflux of contrast into the inferior vena cava during systole.

2D Echo-PLAX View

- On M-mode scan at the ventricular level, there is dilatation of the right ventricular cavity with paradoxical motion of the interventricular septum. The septum moves away from the left ventricle and towards the right ventricle in systole (Fig. 12.19). There is increased amplitude of motion of the RV free wall.

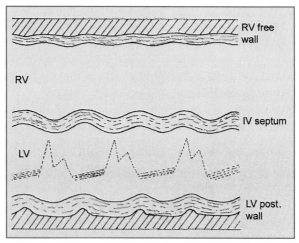

Fig. 12.19: M-mode scan at the ventricular level showing:
    A. Dilatation of the right ventricle
    B. Paradoxical motion of the interventricular septum

- The tricuspid valve can be visualized from the right ventricular inflow tract view, by slight medial angulation from the long axis view. On M-mode scan at this level, there is exaggerated TV leaflet excursion and quick diastolic TV closure due to rapid diastolic filling (short deceleration time).

2-D Echo-PSAX View

- The tricuspid valve can also be visualized from the short-axis view at the aortic valve level. It may reveal the underlying cause of TR such as rheumatic thickening, leaflet prolapse, flail leaflet, endocarditis or Ebstein's anomaly.

Colour Flow Mapping

- A regurgitant jet is seen in the right atrium (RA) along the interatrial septum (Fig. 12.20). The extent to which

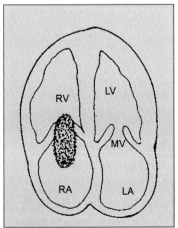

Fig. 12.20: Colour flow mapping from the apical 4-chamber view showing a TR jet in the right atrium

the TR jet fills the RA cavity indicates the severity of TR as shown in Table 12.5.

Table 12.5: Assessment of TR severity by colour flow mapping	
TR severity	*% of RA area*
Mild	< 25
Moderate	25-50
Severe	> 50

- The width of the TR jet correlates with the degree of regurgitation. A broad colour flow signal (wide jet) represents severe TR.

Doppler Echo

- On CW Doppler, scanning the right atrium can pick up the TR jet (Fig. 12.21). The velocity exceeds 2 m/sec and rises further during inspiration. Severity of TR is not related to the velocity but to the density of the signal.
- A flow profile of high velocity with quick acceleration and rapid deceleration is an indicator of severe TR. It

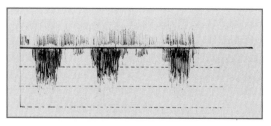

Fig. 12.21: Continuous-wave (CW) Doppler from the apical 4-chamber view showing a TR flow signal in the right atrium

occurs due to rapid equalization of RV and RA pressures: the "common-chamber effect".

- On PW Doppler, mapping progressively deeper into the right atrium (RA) till flow is not seen, can quantify the severity of TR as shown in Table 12.6.

Table 12.6: Assessment of TR severity by PW Doppler

TR severity	Depth of flow in RA
Mild	< 1 cm
Moderate	1-3 cm
Severe	> 3 cm

- On PW Doppler, with the sample volume in the inferior vena cava, retrograde systolic flow (from right atrium to IVC) may be detected.

Doppler Calculations

- When tricuspid regurgitation is secondary to right ventricular enlargement and dilatation of the TV annulus, as it often is, the transtricuspid flow velocity (Vmax) is used to calculate the pulmonary artery pressure (Fig. 12.22). The following Doppler calculations are employed:

RV pressure (RVP)– = Pressure gradient (PG)
RA pressure (RAP)   across TV
$RVP = PG + RAP$ = $4 Vmax^2 + RAP$
RV pressure = Pulmonary artery pressure (if no pulmonary stenosis)

Therefore, PA pressure = $4Vmax^2 + RAP$
If the Vmax is > 2.5 m/sec and RAP is > 5 mm,

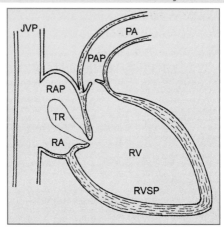

Fig. 12.22: The principle of estimating pulmonary artery pressure from the tricuspid regurgitant jet

PA pressure $= 4 \times (2.5)^2 + >5$ mm
                      $= 4 \times 6.25 + >5$ mm
                      $= 25 + >5$ mm
                      $= >30$ mmHg
(see Pulmonary Hypertension)

Causes of TR

The causes of TR can be classified as primary diseases of the tricuspid valve and TR secondary to dilatation of the TV annulus. Primary causes of TR are similar to those of mitral regurgitation. Secondary TR is due to enlargement of the right ventricle.

Primary Causes

- Rheumatic heart disease
- Tricuspid valve prolapse

- Flail tricuspid leaflet
- Right-sided endocarditis
- Papillary muscle dysfunction
- Connective tissue disorders
- Carcinoid syndrome
- Ebstein's anomaly

Secondary Causes

- Pulmonary hypertension due to:
  — Eisenmenger's reaction
  — Rheumatic mitral disease
  — Chronic cor pulmonale
  — Primary pulmonary hypertension
- Cardiomyopathy:
  — Dilated CMP
  — Restrictive CMP
- Right ventricular volume overload:
  — Pulmonary valve disease (PS)
  — Septal defect (ASD, VSD)

EBSTEIN'S ANOMALY

Echo Features of Ebstein's Anomaly

2-D Echo AP4CH View

- There is downward displacement of the tricuspid valve into the body of the right ventricle towards the RV apex. The mitral and tricuspid valve planes are thus offset. The septal TV leaflet is attached to the IV septum, 10 mm or more inferior to the anterior mitral leaflet (Fig. 12.23).

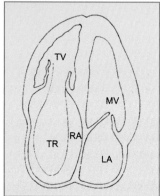

Fig. 12.23: Echo features of Ebstein's anomaly:
A. Downward displacement of tricuspid valve,
B. Enlargement of the right atrium,
C. A tricuspid regurgitant jet

- The anterior tricuspid leaflet (ATL) is large and shows wide excursion, often with a whip-like motion.
- The right ventricle is dilated and hyperkinetic due to volume overload.
- The right atrium is enlarged because of the tricuspid valvular abnormality as well as due to "atrialization" of the upper part of right ventricle.

PLAX View and M-Mode

- Because of downward displacement of the tricuspid valve, there is simultaneous recording of the mitral and tricuspid valves (MV and TV) at the same position.
- Closure of the TV is delayed and occurs more than 60 millisec after MV closure.

PSAX View

- Due to inferior displacement of the TV, it is shifted clockwise from the normal 9 o'clock position to the 11 o'clock position.

AORTIC STENOSIS

Causes of AS

Valvular AS

- Rheumatic AS   rheumatic heart disease
- Calcific AS   senile degenerative valve
- Congenital AS   bicuspid aortic valve.

Subvalvular AS

- Subaortic AS   discrete membrane /ring
- Tunnel-type AS   diffuse muscular narrowing
- IHSS/HOCM   hypertrophic cardiomyopathy.

Supravalvular AS

- William's syndrome   discrete membrane
- Hour-glass AS   focal narrowing

Echo Features of AS

2-D Echo PLAX View

- The aortic valve leaflets are thickened due to fibrosis with or without calcification, in valvular AS. In rheumatic AS, the process starts in the leaflets with fusion of commissures followed by secondary calcification of leaflets and annulus (Fig. 12.24A). In calcific AS, the process starts with calcification of the annulus and progresses medially to involve the leaflets (Fig. 12.24B). In bicuspid aortic valve, calcification is observed only in the late stages of the disease and not to begin with.

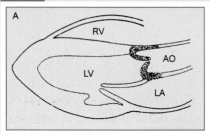

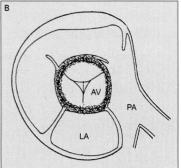

Fig. 12.24: Calcification of the aortic valve seen on echo:
A PLAX view—calcification of leaflets
B PSAX view—calcification of annulus

- There is reduced excursion of aortic leaflets with restricted opening of the aortic valve. Due to fusion at the leaflet tips and free motion of the leaflet bodies, there is systolic doming. This is a characteristic feature of rheumatic AS. Leaflet excursion is normal in a bicuspid aortic valve unless it is heavily calcified.
- In a bicuspid aortic valve, there may be prolapse of the right coronary cusp into the left ventricular outflow tract (LVOT) during diastole.
- In valvular AS, there is poststenotic dilatation of the proximal aorta (normal aortic root diameter is 20-37 mm). This is due to the high velocity jet through the narrow and distorted valve, impinging on the wall of the ascending aorta.

- In supravalvular AS, a thin linear echo (discrete membrane) extends inwards from the aortic wall. With an hour-glass AS, there is a gradual decrease in aortic root diameter during superoinferior angulation of the transducer.

- In membranous subaortic AS, there is a linear echo (discrete membrane) in the LV outflow tract, between the IV septum and the AML of mitral valve. The linear echo is proximal and parallel to the aortic valve sometimes with a T-artefact at its free edge.

- In tunnel-type subaortic AS, the left ventricular outflow tract (LVOT) appears narrower than the aortic root.

- In long-standing AS, there is often evidence of left ventricular hypertrophy (LVH) due to left ventricular systolic (pressure) overload. There is thickening of the IV septum and LV posterior wall which exceeds 12 mm. This leads to a small LV cavity with good LV systolic function. In LVH, the left ventricular mass exceeds 134 grams/m^2 in men and 110 grams/m^2 in females. In later stages of AS, especially with associated aortic regurgitation (AR), there is LV dilatation with LV systolic dysfunction (see Ventricular Dysfunction). This clinical course of LV hypertrophy followed by LV dilatation is also observed in systemic hypertension and coarctation of aorta (see Systemic Hypertension).

2-D Echo PSAX View

- On short-axis view at aortic valve level, there is leaflet thickening, reduced excursion, calcification and a small AV lumen.

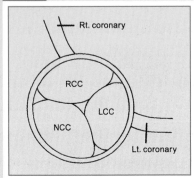

Fig. 12.25: Normal triradiate anatomy of aortic cusps seen on short axis view:
RCC—right coronary cusp
LCC—left coronary cusp
NCC—non coronary cusp

- A bicuspid valve can be identified from this view. It results from failure of two of the aortic cusps to separate during embryologic development. Therefore, there are 2 cusps and 2 commissures while the 3rd commissure (between right and left cusps) is replaced by a raphe. Thus, there is distortion of the normal triradiate anatomy of aortic valve cusps (Fig. 12.25).

M-mode AV Level

- Normally, on M-mode scan from PLAX view at the aortic valve level, the aortic cusps form a central closure line in diastole. In systole they open to form a box-like opening or parallelogram shape. The normal aortic cusp separation in systole is 15-26 mm.
- In AS, the closure line and box-like opening are replaced by multiple thick dense echoes in the aortic root throughout the cardiac cycle. Individual cusps and their motion are hard to dicipher (Fig. 12.26).
- Due to restricted leaflet excursion, the size of box-like opening of the AV is reduced. The severity of AS

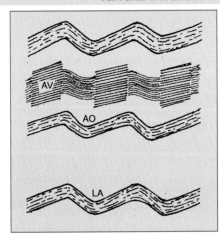

Fig. 12.26: M-mode scan of aortic valve showing multiple thick dense echoes in the aortic root

can be gauged from the size of AV opening as shown in Table 12.7.

Table 12.7: Assessment of AS severity from AV opening	
Severity of AS	*Size of AV opening*
Mild	13-15 mm
Moderate	8-12 mm
Severe	< 8 mm

- In subvalvular AS, there is early or midsystolic closure of the aortic valve (Fig. 12.27), particularly of the right coronary cusp, with fluttering of the cusp in rest of systole. The subvalvular high velocity draws the cusps into a semiclosed position by the Venturi effect.
- The closure line of the aortic valve in diastole is normally central and equidistant from the anterior and posterior aortic walls (Fig. 12.28). In bicuspid aortic

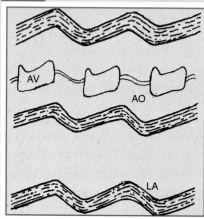

Fig. 12.27: M-mode scan of aortic valve showing midsystolic closure in subvalvular aortic stenosis

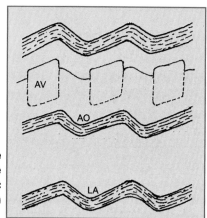

Fig. 12.28: M-mode scan of aortic valve showing an eccentric diastolic closure line in bicuspid aortic valve

valve, the closure line is eccentric or off-centre and closer to one of the aortic walls. Eccentricity of the closure line is expressed by the aortic eccentricity index (see below). An aortic eccentricity index greater than 1.5 is significant.

$$\text{Aortic eccentricity index} = \frac{\text{Aortic root diameter} \times 0.5}{\text{Distance between closure line and nearest aortic wall}}$$

Colour Flow Mapping

- In the AP5CH view, there is a colour flow jet in the proximal aorta (Fig. 12.29). The width of the jet approximates the size of the AV orifice. The location of the jet is below or above the aortic valve level in subvalvular and supravalvular AS respectively.

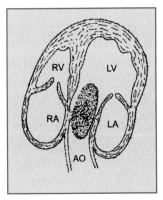

Fig. 12.29: Colour flow mapping from the apical 5-chamber view showing a jet in the proximal aorta

Doppler Echo

- The normal peak aortic systolic outflow velocity ranges from 0.9 to 1.8 m/sec with a mean of 1.3 m/sec. In AS it exceeds 2 m/sec (Fig. 12.30). It can be picked up from the apical view, the right parasternal view and the suprasternal window. Multiple windows need to be examined to obtain parallelism between

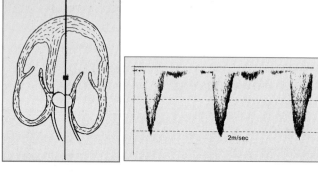

Fig. 12.30: Pulsed-wave (PW) Doppler from the apical 5-chamber view showing increased systolic velocity across the aortic valve

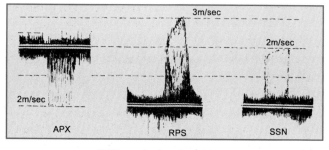

APX—apical 5-chamber view
RPS—right parasternal window
SSN—suprasternal notch.

Fig. 12.31: Continuous wave (CW) Doppler from multiple echo windows in aortic stenosis with a peak velocity of 3 m/sec

the Doppler beam and aortic flow and thus to estimate the true peak aortic velocity (Vmax) (Fig. 12.31).

• The peak velocity is obtained below or above the aortic valve level in subvalvular and supravalvular AS respectively.

- The peak instantaneous transvalvular pressure gradient can be estimated by the following calculations:

Peak PG = $4V^2max - 4V^2_{LVOT} = 4 (V^2max - V^2_{LVOT})$

Vmax = peak AV velocity by CW Doppler

V_{LVOT} = peak LVOT velocity by PW Doppler

V_{LVOT} can be ignored if it is <1 as in moderate to severe AS since V_{LVOT} occurs later in systole. V_{LVOT} should be taken into account in mild AS and in the presence of AR or else a falsely high pressure gradient may be calculated.

Remember, this peak instantaneous pressure gradient is different from the peak-to-peak pressure gradient obtained during cardiac catheterization.

- The severity of AS correlates with peak aortic velocity and transvalvular pressure gradient as shown in Table 12.8.

Table 12.8: Assessment of AS severity from peak velocity and pressure gradient		
Severity of AS	*Peak velocity (m/sec)*	*Pressure gradient (mmHg)*
Mild	1-2	< 20
Moderate	2-4	20-64
Severe	> 4	> 64

Doppler Calculations

- The transaortic pressure gradient depends upon variables including heart rate, stroke volume and the parallelism obtained between the Doppler beam and blood flow. Therefore, it may not be a true indicator

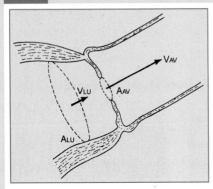

Fig. 12.32: The principle of calculating aortic valve orifice area using the continuity equation

of the severity of valvular stenosis. Calculation of the aortic valve orifice area using the continuity equation is therefore more accurate. The continuity equation relies on the simple principle that the volume of blood leaving the LV is equal to the volume of blood crossing the AV (Fig. 12.32). The aortic valve area is calculated as follows:

$$V_{max} \text{ AV} \times \text{AV area} = V_{max} \text{ LVOT} \times \text{LVOT area}$$

$$\text{AV area} = \frac{V_{max} \text{ LVOT}}{V_{max} \text{ AV}} \times \text{LVOT area}$$

$$\text{LVOT area} = \pi (D/2)^2$$

$$= \frac{22}{7} \times \frac{D^2}{4} = 0.786 \times D^2$$

$$D = \text{diameter of aortic annulus}$$

$$\text{Thus AV area} = \frac{V_{max} \text{ LVOT}}{V_{max} \text{ AV}} \times 0.786 \times D^2$$

This equation is not helpful if V_{max} AV is less than 2 m/sec.

- The severity of AS correlates with the aortic valve area as shown in Table 12.9.

Table 12.9: Assessment of AS severity from AV area	
Severity of AS	AV area (cm²)
Mild	1.5-2.5
Moderate	0.75-1.5
Severe	< 0.75

Pitfalls in the Diagnosis of AS

- Once the aortic valve is heavily calcified, it is difficult to visualize the leaflets separately. In that case, it is not possible to differentiate between a tricuspid and bicuspid aortic valve as also between rheumatic and calcific AS.
- In a condition referred to as aortic sclerosis in the elderly, there is calcification of the aortic valve without any restriction of valve opening or leaflet excursion.
- Abnormalities of leaflets such as thickening, doming, fixity and calcification are not observed in supra-valvular or subvalvular types of AS. Clinically, an ejection click and systolic thrill are only observed in valvular AS.
- The development of left ventricular hypertrophy (LVH) in AS is similar to that observed in other conditions causing LV pressure overload such as systemic hypertension and coarctation of aorta (see Systemic Hypertension).
- Reduction in size of box-like opening of aortic valve is a feature of moderate to severe AS. It is also observed in other low cardiac output states.
- Reverberation of echoes from a heavily calcified valve may cause an apparent increase in cusp thickness.

In that case, the severity of AS is likely to be over-estimated.

- Besides subvalvular AS, midsystolic closure of the aortic valve is observed in HOCM (hypertrophic cardiomyopathy) with dynamic LVOT obstruction. It is also seen in moderate to severe mitral regurgitation (MR) and ventricular septal defect (VSD) where part of the LV stroke volume enters the left atrium and right ventricle respectively.

- Besides in bicuspid aortic valve, an eccentric diastolic closure line may also be observed with a tricuspid aortic valve when there is a subaortic VSD and prolapse of the right coronary cusp into the LVOT.

- In subvalvular and supravalvular AS, on colour flow mapping and on CW Doppler, the colour jet and pressure gradient are observed below and above the aortic valve level respectively.

- The transaortic peak velocity and thus the pressure gradient depends upon the degree of parallelism obtained between the Doppler beam and the aortic flow. They may be underestimated if the Doppler beam is not in line with the flow or if the velocity jet is eccentric in direction.

- The transvalvular pressure gradient depends upon the heart rate and stroke volume. It tends to be overestimated in bradycardia (longer LV filling time) and high cardiac output (aortic regurgitation). It tends to be underestimated in tachycardia (shorter LV filling time) and low cardiac output (LV dysfunction).

- A high velocity jet in the left ventricular outflow tract (LVOT) may be observed in hypertrophic cardiomyo-pathy (HOCM) at the point of contact between the anterior mitral leaflet (AML) and the interventricular septum (IVS). This is obtained on PW Doppler with the sample volume in the LVOT proximal to the aortic valve (see Cardiomyopathies).

- In the presence of AS, LV ejection fraction (LVEF) may be low despite normal LV contractility. This is because the left ventricle has to overcome a high transaortic resistance during ejection. After aortic valve replacement, the LVEF is likely to rise.
- The severity of AS is not related to the loudness of the ejection systolic murmur. Turbulent flow across a mildly stenosed valve can cause a loud murmur while marked restriction to blood flow across a severely stenosed valve can cause a soft murmur.

Indications for Surgical Intervention in AS

A stenotic aortic valve needs repair/replacement in the following situations:
- Severe AS (PG > 64 mmHg ; AV area < 0.75 cm^2)
- Moderate AS with symptoms (angina, syncope)
- Moderate AS without symptoms but high activity level.
- Moderate AS with other cardiac surgery (e.g. CABG)
- Moderate to severe AS with LV systolic dysfunction.

AORTIC REGURGITATION

Causes of AR

Valvular AR

- Rheumatic heart disease
- Congenital heart disease
  a. bicuspid aortic valve
  b. subvalvular aortic stenosis

- Connective tissue disorders
  e.g. SLE, rheumatoid arthritis

Aortic Root Dilatation

- Systemic hypertension
- Medial necrosis:
  a. Marfan's Syndrome
  b. Ehlers-Danlos Syndrome
- Aortitis:
  a. tubercular
  b. syphilitic (rare)
- Inflammatory diseases
  a. Reiter's Syndrome
  b. ankylosing spondylitis.

Acute AR

- Aortic dissection
- Bacterial endocarditis
- Chest wall trauma

Echo Features of AR

M-mode LV Level

- The left ventricle is dilated and hyperkinetic due to volume overload (Fig. 12.33). Similar overloading of the left ventricle is observed in mitral regurgitation. The motion of the IV septum and the LV posterior wall is exaggerated.

2-D Echo PLAX View

- The aortic root is dilated (normal size 20-37 mm) more so if the cause of AR is disease of the aorta

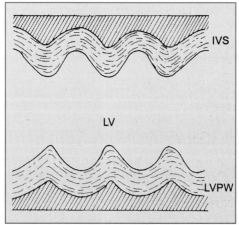

Fig. 12.33: M-mode scan at the ventricular level showing a dilated and hyperkinetic left ventricle with exaggerated motion of the ventricular septum and posterior wall

and less with aortic valvular disease. There may be features of aortic dissection.

• The aortic valve architecture suggests the underlying cause of aortic regurgitation. There may be a bicuspid aortic valve or vegetations on leaflets in endocarditis. Rheumatic AR is suggested by thickened and fibrosed leaflets, non-coaptation of AV cusps and associated mitral valve disease.

M-mode AV level

• There is dilatation of the aortic root.
• The diastolic closure line is eccentric in bicuspid aortic valve
• AR of rheumatic aetiology is often associated with some degree of aortic valve stenosis (AS). There may

be thick dense echoes in the aortic root obscuring the clear outline of cusps.

- Fluttering of an AV cusp in diastole is observed if it has ruptured due to endocarditis. Vegetations may be seen on the leaflet.
- The left atrium may be dilated due to associated mitral valve disease.

M-mode MV Level

- There is fluttering of the anterior mitral leaflet (AML) in diastole, which is sandwiched between the aortic regurgitant flow and the left atrial emptying stream (Fig. 12.34). This is the basis of the Austin-Flint murmur auscultated in AR.

  Note
    1. There may also be fluttering of the interventricular septum (IVS), depending upon the direction of the regurgitant jet
    2. Diastolic flutter of AML is not observed if there is mitral stenosis (thick AML), acute AR (early mitral valve closure) or severe AR (shortened diastole)

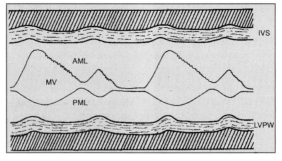

Fig. 12.34: M-mode scan at the mitral valve level showing diastolic fluttering of the anterior mitral leaflet

- Premature closure of the mitral valve (MV) occurs due to rapid completion of diastole especially in acute or severe AR. It indicates an elevated left ventricular end-diastolic pressure (LVEDP)

M-mode LV Dimensions

- The left ventricular internal dimensions in end-diastole and end-systole (LVESD and LVEDD) are increased. Indices of left ventricular function (fractional shortening and ejection fraction) suggest good LV function in early stages of the disease. Later on, there may be severe LV dilatation and systolic dysfunction (see Ventricular Dysfunction). Symptomatic and progressive LV dilatation with an LVESD in excess of 55 mm is an indication for surgical intervention. There is eccentric LV hypertrophy which is inadequate for the degree of LV dilatation (see Systemic Hypertension)
- There may be diastolic fluttering of the interventricular septum (IVS) if the regurgitant jet is directed towards it and not towards the anterior mitral leaflet (AML).

Colour Flow Mapping

- A regurgitant jet is seen entering the left ventricular cavity on PLAX and AP5CH views (Fig. 12.35). The width of the AR jet in the left ventricular outflow tract (LVOT) just below the aortic valve indicates the severity of AR as shown in Table 12.10.
- The extent of the AR jet entry into the LV cavity can also indicate the severity of AR as shown in Table 12.11.

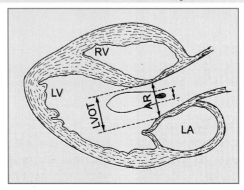

Fig. 12.35: The ratio between the width of AR jet and diameter of LV outflow tract indicates the severity of regurgitation

Table 12.10: Assessment of AR severity from width of jet	
AR severity	*Jet: LVOT width*
Mild	< 25 %
Moderate	25-50%
Severe	> 50%

Table 12.11: Assessment of AR severity from depth of jet	
AR severity	*Extent of jet*
+1	only in LVOT
+2	up to tip of AML
+3	up to 1/2 of tip-apex
+4	up to apex of LV

Doppler Echo

- On PW Doppler using the AP5CH view, with the sample volume just proximal to the aortic valve, the

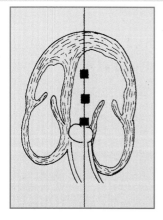

Fig. 12.36: Pulsed-wave (PW) Doppler recording progressively deep into the left ventricle indicates the severity of regurgitation

AR signal can be detected (Fig. 12.36). Since the signal is towards the transducer, it is above the baseline. However, because the AR velocity usually exceeds 2 m/sec, aliasing does occur. In that case, CW Doppler is more useful as it can measure a higher velocity without aliasing and the signal is only above the baseline.

- On PW Doppler, mapping progressively deeper into the left ventricle till flow is not seen can quantify the severity of AR as shown in Table 12.12.

Table 12.12: Assessment of AR severity by Doppler	
AR severity	*Depth of flow in LV*
Mild	within LVOT
Moderate	up to MV (mid LV)
Severe	up to LV apex

- On PW Doppler, with the sample volume in the aortic arch from the suprasternal window, diastolic flow reversal of high velocity and long duration indicates the presence of severe AR.

- CW Doppler can detect the high velocity AR signal without aliasing. However, severity of AR is not only related to the velocity but also to the density or intensity of the flow signal. A dense or intense signal indicates that greater volume of blood is moving at a given velocity.

Doppler Calculations

- The severity of AR can be gauged from the rate of deceleration of the AR velocity profile. A rapid deceleration rate (steep fall) indicates rapid equalization of the pressure difference between the aorta and the LV cavity and therefore severe AR. In other words, steeper the slope, more severe is the AR. Deceleration rate is expressed in metres/second per second or m/sec^2 (Fig. 12.37).

  Another way to express this principle is by measuring the time taken for the peak pressure gradient across the aortic valve to drop to half of its original value, which is the pressure half-time. The quicker the equalization of the pressure difference between the aorta and LV (short pressure half-time), more severe is the AR. Pressure half-time is expressed in milliseconds or millisec.

- The severity of AR correlates with the deceleration rate and pressure half-time as shown in Table 12.13.

Pitfalls in the Diagnosis of AR

- M-mode and 2-D echo cannot directly diagnose AR but can indicate the cause and the effects of AR on

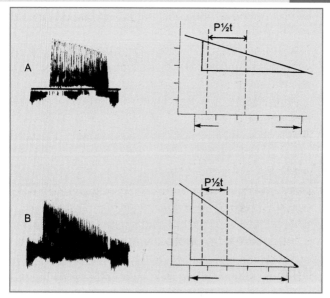

Fig. 12.37: Relationship between rate of velocity deceleration
and severity of aortic regurgitation:
A. flat slope: mild AR,
B. steep slope: severe AR

Table 12.13: Assessment of AR severity from rate of deceleration of velocity

Severity of AR	Deceleration rate (m/sec²)	Pressure half-time (millisec)
Mild	< 2	> 400
Moderate	2-3	300-400
Severe	> 3	< 300

the aortic root and left ventricle. They can pick up
aortic root dilatation, aortic valve abnormalities and
left ventricular dilatation. Colour flow mapping and

Doppler echo can not only detect AR but also assess its severity.

- The diagnosis of AR may be straightforward but assessment of its severity is complex and requires several echo criteria. Even then, distinguishing mild from moderate AR may be particularly difficult while severe AR is readily picked up.

- The AR jet may be underestimated or even altogether missed if it is eccentric. This error can be avoided by scanning the entire left ventricular outflow tract by placing the sample volume of PW Doppler in different positions from different echo views.

- The width and length of the AR jet provides quantitative information about the severity of AR. This is not a fool-proof method since the narrow jet of mild AR may extend deep into the LV while a broad jet of severe AR may not extend far if it is eccentric.

- In acute AR due to dissection, endocarditis or trauma, there is no time for left ventricular dilatation to develop. A small-volume high-velocity AR jet is observed with an acute rise of left ventricular end-diastolic pressure (LVEDP) and pulmonary oedema.

- The AR jet may be difficult to differentiate from the jet of mitral stenosis, particularly in the AP5CH view. The matter is further complicated by the fact that AR and MS often coexist in rheumatic heart disease. On PW Doppler, the 2 jets can be differentiated by mapping the LV outflow tract and MV area separately. On CW Doppler, AR shows a high velocity (> 2 m/sec) signal throughout diastole while MS shows a lower velocity (usually < 2 m/sec) signal in mid-diastole (after isovolumic relaxation).

Criteria for Severe AR

- Colour flow jet width: LVOT width >50%
- Diastolic flow reversal in the aortic arch
- Rapid AR velocity decay (P½ t < 300 msec).
- Dense flow signal on CW Doppler
- Flow up to LV apex on PW Doppler
- Left ventricular volume overload

Indications for Surgical Intervention in AR

A regurgitant aortic valve needs surgical repair or replacement in the following situations:

- Moderate to severe AR with severe symptoms (effort intolerance)
- Asymptomatic severe AR with LV dysfunction (LVEF < 50%)
- Asymptomatic severe AR with LV dilatation (LVESD > 55 mm)
- Acute AR with haemodynamic compromise (e.g. aortic dissection)

PULMONARY STENOSIS

Causes of PS

Valvular PS

- Congenital PS:
  - a. isolated (commonest)
  - b. rubella syndrome
- Acquired PS:
  - a rheumatic heart disease (rare)
  - b. carcinoid syndrome

Subvalvular PS

Isolated (rare)
With VSD, TOF, TGV

Supravalvular PS

Rubella syndrome
With supra-aortic AS

Echo Features of PS

2-D Echo PSAX View

- In valvular PS, the pulmonary valve leaflets are thickened and calcified. There is systolic doming of leaflets with reduced excursion and restricted opening of the pulmonary valve.
- There may be poststenotic dilatation of the pulmonary artery. This is because of the high velocity jet through the narrow valve, impinging on the wall of the pulmonary artery.
- In subvalvular PS, the right ventricular outflow tract (RVOT) appears narrower than the pulmonary root. Alternatively, a discrete muscular band is seen in the RVOT. The pulmonary valve leaflets are normal and usually there is no poststenotic dilatation of the pulmonary artery.
- In supravalvular PS, a discrete shelf-like band may be seen in the pulmonary artery. Alternatively, a long stenotic tunnel-like area is observed distal to the pulmonary valve.

M-mode PV Level

- In valvular PS, besides thickening of the PV cusps, there is a prominent 'a' wave on the pulmonary valve trace. This occurs because of doming of the pulmonary leaflets.

- In subvalvular (infundibular) PS, there is premature closure of the PV in midsystole with fluttering of the PV leaflets in the rest of systole.
- In supravalvular PS, scanning at the PV level reveals no abnormality.

2-D Echo PLAX View

- The effect of PS on the right ventricle is the same, irrespective of the site of obstruction whether it is valvular, subvalvular or supravalvular stenosis.
- There is evidence of right ventricular systolic (pressure) overload. This causes RV free wall thickness > 5 mm with or without RV dilatation > 23 mm and paradoxical motion of the interventricular septum (IVS)

Colour Flow Mapping

- There is a colour flow jet in the proximal pulmonary artery in valvular PS (Fig. 12.38). The width of the jet approximates the size of the PV orifice. The location of jet is below or above the pulmonary valve level in subvalvular and supravalvular PS respectively.

Doppler Echo

- The normal peak pulmonary systolic outflow velocity ranges from 0.5 to 1.0 m/sec with a mean of 0.75 m/sec. In PS it exceeds 1 m/sec (Fig. 12.39). In valvular PS, the peak velocity indicates the pressure gradient

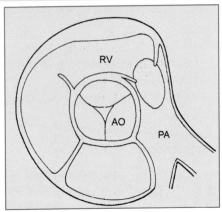

Fig. 12.38: Colour flow mapping from the short-axis view showing a jet in the proximal pulmonary artery

across the pulmonary valve. In subvalvular or supravalvular PS, the peak velocity is obtained below or above the PV. Accordingly, it indicates the pressure gradient across the site of narrowing.

Severity of PS

The severity of PS correlates with the pressure gradient across the valve and estimated valve area as shown in Table 12.14.

Table 12.14: Assessment of PS severity from pressure gradient		
Severity of PS	Valve area (cm²)	Pressure gradient (mm Hg)
Mild	> 1.0	< 25
Moderate	0.5-1.0	25-40
Severe	< 0.5	> 40

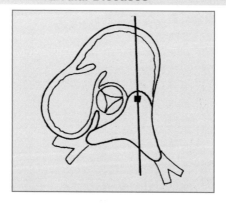

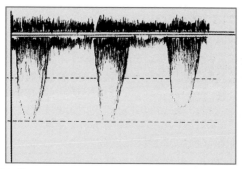

Fig. 12.39: Pulsed-wave (PW) Doppler from the short-axis view showing increased systolic outflow velocity across the pulmonary valve

PULMONARY REGURGITATION

Causes of PR

Primary Causes

PR is rarely due to primary causes:
- rheumatic heart disease

- right-sided endocarditis
- carcinoid syndrome

Congenital Causes

PR is sometimes congenital in origin:
- pulmonary valve atresia
- subvalvular PS.

Iatrogenic Causes

PR is occasionally induced during catheterization:
- surgery
- valvotomy
- angiography

Secondary Cause

PR is most commonly secondary to:
- pulmonary hypertension.

Echo Features of PR

2-D Echo PLAX View

- The right ventricle is dilated and hyperkinetic due to volume overload. The motion of the RV free wall is exaggerated. The dimension of the RV often exceeds 23 mm. There is paradoxical motion of the interventricular septum (IVS).

2-D Echo PSAX View

- The pulmonary artery is dilated and its diameter exceeds that of the aorta (20-37 mm).

- The PV leaflets are thick and immobile in rheumatic heart disease and carcinoid syndrome. Vegetations are observed in endocarditis. In PV atresia, pulmonary cusps are replaced by a ridge of tissue.

M-Mode PV Level

- In valvular PS and PR, there is a prominent 'a' wave on the PV trace.
- In subvalvular PS and PR there is systolic fluttering of PV leaflets
- In PR due to pulmonary hypertension, the 'a' wave is absent.

Colour Flow Mapping

- A regurgitant jet is visualized in the right ventricular outflow tract (RVOT) just below the pulmonary valve (Fig. 12.40).

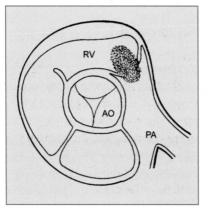

Fig. 12.40: Colour flow mapping from the short-axis view showing a regurgitant jet in the RV outflow tract

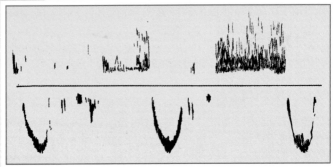

Fig. 12.41: Continuous wave (CW) Doppler from the short-axis view showing a "bullet-shaped" flow signal in the right ventricular outflow tract (RVOT)

- The width of the PR jet at the PV level indicates the severity of PR.
- Severity of PR is also indicated by the extent to which the PR jet enters the RV cavity.

Doppler Echo

- On CW Doppler, a dense and intense flow signal is detected.
- A short deceleration time (rapid pressure fall) with a steep slope of the CW Doppler signal correlates with the severity of PR (Fig. 12.41).
- CW Doppler may inadvertantly detect nearby coronary sinus flow due to its inability to localize the flow signal.
- On PW Doppler, mapping progressively deeper into the right ventricle till flow is not seen can quantify the severity of PR. A jet extending lower down from the pulmonary valve indicates severe PR.

CHAPTER THIRTEEN

PERICARDIAL DISEASES

Clinically important diseases of the pericardium are:
1. Pericardial effusion
2. Cardiac tamponade
3. Constrictive pericarditis

PERICARDIAL EFFUSION

The space between 2 layers of the pericardium normally contains less than 50 ml fluid. Excessive accumulation of this fluid is called pericardial effusion.

Echo Features of Pericardial Effusion

Pericardial effusion creates an echo-free space posteriorly between the left ventricular posterior wall and pericardium and anteriorly between the right ventricle free wall and the chest wall. Posterior accumulation of fluid precedes collection of fluid anteriorly (Fig. 13.1).

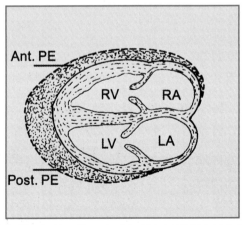

Fig. 13.1: Illustrative figure showing anterior and posterior echo-free space around the heart due to pericardial effusion (PE)

Quantification of Effusion

The quantity of pericardial fluid can be gauged from the width of the echo-free space on M-mode scan from the PLAX view. This is shown in Table 13.1.

Table 13.1: Estimating quantity of pericardial effusion from width of echo-free space			
Amount	Volume	Posterior space	Anterior space
Small	< 100 ml	< 1 cm	—
Moderate	100-300 ml	1-2 cm	< 1 cm
Large	> 300 ml	> 2 cm	> 1 cm

A more accurate method is to use planimetry (area estimation) function of the echo machine soft-ware. A still 2-D image of an apical 4-chamber view is taken and the following tracings are taken:

A : Around the pericardium [Volume of heart + pericardium]

B : Around the heart [Volume of heart]

Volume of pericardial effusion = A minus B.

Causes of Pericardial Effusion

- Infections   -   viral, bacterial, tubercular
- Malignancies   -   metastasis, haematogenous
- Trauma   -   accidental, surgical
- Auto-immune   -   rheumatoid arthritis, SLE
- Metabolic   -   uraemia, myxoedema
- Toxic   -   drug-induced, radiation.
- Infarction   -   post-MI syndrome
                                  (Dressler's syndrome)

Judging Cause of Effusion from Echo

- Transudate   -   sonolucent echo-free fluid
- Sanguinous   -   high echo-density of fluid.
- Tubercular   -   fibrinous strands in effusion
- Malignant   -   echo-dense areas deforming smoothness of pericardium

Pitfalls in the Diagnosis of Effusion

False Negative

A pericardial effusion may be missed on echo if:
- it is loculated and out of path of the echo-beam
- the echo-machine is on a high-gain setting
- the cardiac image is large and extends beyond the far border of the screen.

False Positive

A pericardial effusion may be falsely diagnosed if:
- there is an echo-free space behind the posterior wall due to one of the following:
  - large left atrium
  - descending thoracic aorta
  - aneurysm of posterior wall
  - pericardial cyst/fat pad
- calcified mitral annulus or prominent papillary muscle is mistaken for the left ventricular posterior wall and the latter mimics a pericardial effusion.

  Note: the left ventricular posterior wall should thicken in systole.

Differentiation from Thickened Pericardium

If the pericardium is thickened or there is an organized exudate, it can be differentiated from an effusion by the following criteria:
- increasing gain-settings of the machine reveals linear pericardial echoes.
- the thickened pericardium retains its parallelity to the epicardial surface.
- width of the thickened pericardium remains the same irrespective of the stage in cardiac cycle, phase of respiration and body posture.

Differentiation from Pleural Effusion

A pericardial effusion sometimes need to be differentiated from a left pleural effusion. Unlike a pleural effusion, the echo-free space of a pericardial effusion:
- terminates abruptly at the A-V groove
- does not extend behind descending aorta
- is never more than 4cm in width.

Note: If a pericardial effusion coexists with a pleural effusion, a linear echo (thick pericardium) separates the two effusions (Fig. 13.2).

CARDIAC TAMPONADE

Cardiac tamponade is a serious clinical situation in which cardiac function is impaired due to external pressure exerted on the heart by a pericardial effusion. Tamponade results from a large volume of effusion or a rapidly formation of a small effusion.

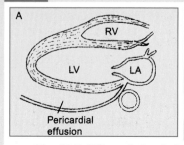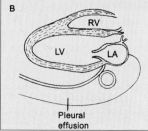

Fig. 13.2: Differentiation between pericardial effusion
(A) and pleural effusion
(B) by 2D Echo-PLAX view

Note: A large effusion can accumulate gradually without causing tamponade if the pericardial sac gets adequate time to stretch itself.

Echo Features of Cardiac Tamponade

- Large volume of pericardial effusion (see above)
- Diastolic collapse of right atrium and right ventricle on M-mode scan. The right ventricular free wall merges with the interventricular septum obliterating the right ventricular cavity (Fig. 13.3).

  Note:
  1. Duration and severity of collapse correlates with the severity of tamponade.
  2. Collapse may be absent if there is right ventricular hypertrophy or if there are pericardial adhesions.
- Swinging heart on 2-D echo with anterior and posterior walls moving in the same direction during most of the cardiac cycle.

  Note: The heart swings because of undulation of chambers caused by displacement of fluid within the

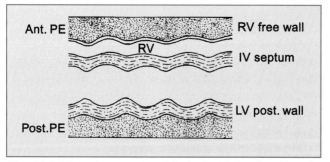

Fig. 13.3: M-mode scan at ventricular level showing diastolic collapse of the right ventricle in a patient of cardiac tamponade

confines of a stretched pericardial sac. Increase in volume of one chamber leads to decrease in volume of the other.

- Exaggerated changes in right and left ventricular dimensions with respiration.

    Note: RV volume increases and LV volume falls during inspiration. The reverse occurs during expiration. On Doppler, exaggerated change is observed in transmitral and transtricuspid flow velocities.

- Anterior mitral leaflet shows pseudo-SAM and pseudo-MVP. Pseudo-systolic anterior motion (SAM) occurs during anterior swing of the heart while pseudo-mitral valve prolapse (MVP) occurs during posterior swing of the heart.

Echo and Pericardiocentesis

- Echo aids in safe performance of therapeutic echo-guided needle aspiration of pericardial fluid: pericardiocentesis.

- Relief of tamponade is a life-saving procedure the success of which can be gauged by post-procedure repeat echo.
- After pericardiocentesis, RV diastolic collapse reverses sooner than RA collapse. Therefore, RA collapse may be a more sensitive indicator of impending tamponade.

CONSTRICTIVE PERICARDITIS

In pericardial constriction, the pericardium becomes thick, rigid and often calcific. Constrictive pericarditis limits the expansion of the ventricles and thus impairs diastolic filling.

ECHO Features of Constrictive Pericarditis

- On M-mode and 2-D echo, the thickened pericardium appears as a dark thick echo line or as multiple parallel lines depending upon the gain setting of the echo machine. Calcification of the pericardium casts a bright reflection.
- There is abrupt anterior motion of interventricular septum (IVS) in diastole with paradoxical systolic motion.
- Rapid early diastolic descent of left ventricular posterior wall (LVPW) with flattening of LVPW motion in mid and late diastole is observed.

  Note: This diastolic filling pattern is a reflection of the dip and plateau pattern (square-root sign) of the left ventricular pressure trace. On the JVP it is reflected as a prominent 'X' descent.

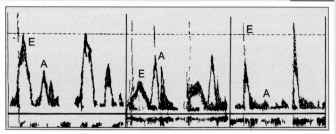

Fig. 13.4: Mitral inflow spectral space on PW Doppler showing a large E wave, rapid deceleration and a small A wave C in a patient of constrictive pericarditis. A similar picture is observed in restrictive cardiomyopathy

- The inferior vena cava is dilated without an inspiratory reduction in its diameter, due to a raised systemic venous pressure.
- On abdominal sonography, there is hepatomegaly, dilatation of hepatic veins, splenomegaly and ascites.
- On Doppler echo, the mitral valve inflow spectral trace reflects abnormal diastolic left ventricular filling of a restrictive pattern. There is increase in early diastolic velocity with rapid deceleration resulting in a large E wave and a small A wave (Fig. 13.4).
- There is exaggerated respiratory variation of mitral valve (MV) and tricuspid valve (TV) inflow. MV E wave amplitude decreases by > 25% on inspiration and TV E wave decreases by > 25% on expiration.

Differentiation from Restrictive Cardiomyopathy

It is particularly difficult to distinguish constrictive pericarditis from restrictive cardiomyopathy or a

Echo Made Easy

restrictive myocardial dysfunction due to myocardial infiltration (see Cardiomyopathies).

Direct pressure measurements at cardiac catheterization are required to clinch the diagnosis. Nevertheless, subtle differences between the two conditions exist which are enumerated in Table 13.2 below. Differentiation between these two clinical conditions is crucial since it has important management implications.

Table 13.2: Differences between constrictive pericarditis and restrictive cardiomyopathy

	Constrictive pericarditis	Restrictive cardiomyopathy
Pericardium	Thick	Normal
Myocardium	Normal	Thick
Ventricles	Normal	Obliterated
Atria	Normal	Dilated
LV function	Normal	Mildly impaired
MV and TV	Normal	Regurgitation
MV inflow	Abrupt halt	Slow relaxation

CHAPTER FOURTEEN

ENDOCARDIAL
DISEASES

Endocarditis is inflammation of the inner surface of the heart, including the lining of heart valves. Inflammatory and/or infected material accumulates to cause discrete lesions called vegetations. Vegetations are made up of a mixture of infective material, fibrin, platelets and WBCs. Sometimes, endocarditis is due to non-infective diseases.

Causes of Endocarditis

Infective Causes

- Bacterial — Gram-negative bacilli, *Streptococcus*, *Staphylococcus*
- Fungal — *Aspergillus, Candida*
- Others — *Coxiella, Chlamydia*

Non-infective Causes

- Malignant disease — merantic endocarditis
- Collagen disorder — verrucous endocarditis (Libman-Sack's endocardits)
- Rheumatic fever — rheumatic pancarditis.

Cardiac Lesions Predisposing to Endocarditis

Common Lesions

- Valve disease
  —AV: bicuspid, rheumatic
  —MV: regurgitant, prolapse
  —TV: IV drug abuse, cannulation
- Prosthetic valve
  —tissue or mechanical valves

- Congenital disease
  — VSD, PDA, coarctation

Note: Infection at the site of PDA or coarctation is endothelitis and not endocarditis.

Uncommon Lesions

- Pulmonary stenosis
- Atrial septal defect
- HOCM
- AV fistula

Indications for Echo in Endocarditis

- Diagnosis of vegetations
- Detecting predisposing lesion
- Looking for complications
- Evaluating response to treatment
- Timing of surgical intervention

Echo Features of Endocarditis

Detection

Vegetations are detected by M-mode or 2-D techniques as mobile, irregular echo-reflective masses attached to a valve cusp or a cardiac lesion. As a rule, vegetations move in concert with the leaflet and in unison with blood flow. They do not impair valve excursion and are usually seen in one phase of the cardiac cycle, either systole or diastole (Fig. 14.1).

Site

The site of vegetations depends upon the underlying predisposing cardiac lesion. Since they move in unison with blood flow, they are seen in the left atrium in MR, in

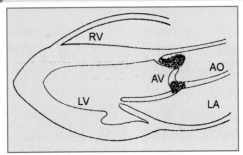

Fig. 14.1: Parasternal long-axis view showing vegetations on the aortic valve leaflets in a case of bacterial endocarditis

the LV outflow tract in AR and on the right ventricular side of a VSD.

Size

The size of vegetations varies from < 1 mm to several cm. Vegetations < 2 mm in size are difficult to visualize. Transesophageal echo vastly improves detection of vegetations. Large vegetations are particularly associated with fungal and tricuspid valve endocarditis. Vegetations shrink as they heal although rapid shrinkage suggests embolization. Mitral valve vegetations are larger the aortic vegetations (see Table 14.2).

Shape

Fresh vegetations are irregular and lumpy but they smoothen as they heal (see Table 14.1). They may be sessile (nodular thickening) or pedunculated.

Echodensity

Fresh vegetations are isoechoic with the leaflet and they get brighter (hyperechoic) as they heal (see Table 14.2).

Mobility

High mobility is observed in large and pedunculated vegetations while mobility is low in small and sessile vegetations. Mitral vegetations are more mobile than aortic vegetations (see Table 14.2) and mobility declines as healing occurs.

Table 14.1: Fresh vegetations versus healed vegetations	
Fresh	*Healed*
Larger	Smaller
Irregular	Smoother
Mobile	Less mobile
Isoechoic	Hyperechoic

Table 14.2: Mitral vegetations versus aortic vegetations	
Mitral	*Aortic*
Larger	Smaller
Mobile	Less mobile
In LA	In LVOT
In systole	In diastole

Differentiation of Vegetations from Other Leaflet Masses

- It may be difficult to differentiate vegetations from other masses on valve leaflets such as nodular degeneration in a myxomatous floppy valve or a valvular thrombus.
- It may also be difficult to diagnose vegetations in the presence of reverberation artefacts caused by a calcific valve annulus or a prosthetic valve.

- A rapid change in echo findings on serial echo-cardiograms with suggestive signs and symptoms favours the diagnosis of endocarditis.

Key Facts about Echo in Endocarditis

- Endocarditis is a clinical diagnosis made on the basis of history, clinical examination, haematological investigations and blood cultures.
- Absence of vegetations on echo does not exclude the diagnosis of endocarditis suspected on clinical grounds.
- It is not possible to distinguish between infective and noninfective vegetations by echocardiography alone.
- Patients of endocarditis without demonstrable vegetations on echo carry a better prognosis. Large vegetations indicate a poorer prognosis with greater likelihood of complications and need for surgical intervention.

DUKE Criteria for Endocarditis

Major

- Persistently positive blood cultures with an organism known to cause endocarditis
- Echo-wise definite vegetation or abscess or new prosthetic dehiscence or new native regurgitation

Minor

- Predisposing heart condition or IV drug use
- Fever with constitutional symptoms e.g. arthralgias, malaise
- Vascular phenomena - emboli, septic infarcts, mycotic aneurysm

- Immunologic: glomerulonephritis, vasculitis, retinal lesion
- Echo consistent with vegetation but no new abnormality.
- Positive blood culture, but not MAJOR criterion
  2 Major criteria or 1 Major and 3 minor criteria are required for the diagnosis of endocarditis.

Detecting Consequences and Complications

- Endocarditis can lead to valve destruction, valvular regurgitation, appearance of a new murmur or change in a preexisting murmur. This occurs due to prolapse, perforation or rupture of a valve leaflet.
- There can be abscess formation around a valve ring or in the interventricular septum which can cause conduction block.
- An aortic root abscess can produce an aneurysm of the sinus of Valsalva or obstruct the coronary ostia.
- A large vegetation (e.g. aortic fungal endocarditis) can obstruct the aortic valve.
- Heart failure may occur due to associated myocarditis, pericardial effusion or acute valvular regurgitation.

Evaluating Response to Treatment

- Healed vegetations differ from fresh ones by being smaller, smoother and hyperechoic (see Table 14.1). Digital processing of the 2-D image showing increasing pixel intensity suggests cure.
- Shrinkage of vegetations alone does not indicate cure while rapid shrinkage suggests embolization. The risk

of embolization persists for upto 6 months after bacteriological cure.

- How often serial echos should be done while the patient is receiving antibiotics is a matter of debate. It is difficult to justify frequent echos unless this will alter clinical management. However, repeat echo should be definitely carried out if there is deterioration in the patient's clinical condition.

Timing of Surgical Intervention

The decision to intervene with a surgical procedure in endocarditis is taken in the following situations:
- Fungal endocarditis
- Failure of antibiotic therapy
- Prosthetic valve endocarditis
- Large vegetation with embolization
- Large vegetation with valve obstruction
- Abscess in aortic root or IV septum
- Valve destruction and regurgitation
- Worsening congestive heart failure
- Sinus of Valsalva aneurysm.

Indications for Transoesophageal Echo

A transthoracic echo needs to be supplemented with a transoesophageal echo in the following situations:
- Normal transthoracic echo with high clinical suspicion
- Poor thoracic window
- Aortic root abscess
- Leaflet perforation or rupture
- Aneurysm sinus of Valsalva
- Prosthetic valve endocarditis.

CHAPTER FIFTEEN

INTRACARDIAC MASSES

CARDIAC TUMOURS

Types of Cardiac Tumours

Secondary Tumours (Majority)

Metastatic: — lung (commonest)
               — breast, kidney, liver
               — melanoma, lymphoma, leukemia

Primary Tumours (Minority)

Benign: — myxoma (commonest)
               — rhabdomyoma, fibroelastoma
               — fibroma, lipoma, angioma
Malignant: — angiosarcoma (commonest)
               — rhabdomyosarcoma
               — fibrosarcoma, liposarcoma

Echo Features of Cardiac Tumours

- 2-D echo shows cardiac tumours as echogenic masses within a cavity of the heart. It tells about the site, size, number, mobility and attachment of tumours to the chamber wall.
- Additional information provided by echo includes obstruction of a valve by the tumour, ventricular dysfunction due to myocardial infiltration and malignant pericardial effusion.

Importance of Echo in Tumours

- Echo is the most important modality for the diagnosis of cardiac tumours.

- Although it gives an indication of the nature of tumour, it cannot readily differentiate between benign and malignant tumours
- As with all echo studies, multiple views should be obtained to delineate the tumour morphology in detail.
- Information about the site, size, mobility, number and attachment of tumours is particularly helpful while planning surgical treatment.
- Vast majority of cardiac tumours are secondary and they are all malignant as they have metastasized. They occur in about 10% of all fatal malignancies. The lung is the most common primary site (30% of cases) because of its close proximity to the heart.
- Myxoma in the left atrium is by far the most common primary cardiac tumour and it is worth knowing about it in greater detail.

LEFT ATRIAL MYXOMA

Clinical Features of LA Myxoma

- Myxoma is a gelatinous and friable cardiac tumour of connective tissue origin.
- It is mostly single and occurs three times more often in the left atrium than in the right atrium
- It is commonly seen in middle-aged women
- Although benign in the neoplastic sense, myxoma is far from being benign in its clinical effects. Effects of myxoma relate to:
  a. local effects like mitral valve obstruction which causes breathlessness and can be fatal when it occurs suddenly.

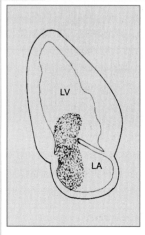

Fig. 15.1: Apical 2-chamber view showing a left atrial myxoma prolapsing through the mitral valve orifice in diastole

  b. distal embolism due to bits of friable tissue breaking away from the main mass

  c. constitutional features such as fever, arthralgias, anaemia and weight loss with an elevated ESR.

Echo Features of LA Myxoma

- On 2-D echo, the myxoma is seen as a mass in the left atrial cavity measuring 2 to 8 cm in size.
- It is usually pedunculated, rarely sessile and attached to the margin of foramen ovale on the interatrial septum
- It is lobulated with a variable echodensity. The centre is echolucent due to necrosis and the periphery is echoreflective due to calcification.
- Most myxomas are mobile and prolapse through the mitral valve inflow orifice in diastole (Fig. 15.1). A myxoma is non-prolapsing if it is either sessile or very large.

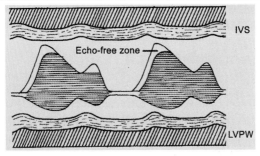

IVS

Echo-free zone

LVPW

Fig. 15.2: M-mode scan of the mitral valve showing cloudy echoes in diastole with an early echo-free zone. This is characteristic of a left atrial myxoma

Differentiation from Mitral Stenosis

- On M-mode scan, myxoma produces cloudy echoes in the mitral inflow in diastole and in the left atrium in systole. Importantly, an echo-free zone is seen in the mitral inflow in early diastole as the valve opening precedes prolapse of the myxoma. This echo-free zone is not observed in mitral stenosis (Fig. 15.2).

- Since the myxoma causes mitral inflow obstruction, there is flattening of the EF slope of anterior mitral leaflet (AML) excursion as observed in mitral stenosis. However, unlike in mitral stenosis, there is no thickening or doming of the AML or paradoxical motion of the posterior mitral leaflet (PML).

- On Doppler echo, the myxoma produces a high velocity signal as does mitral stenosis. The difference in the signal due to myxoma is that it is irregular due to multiple jets around the tumour.

Note: Since the extent of prolapse of the myxoma into the MV inflow varies with body posture, the 2-D,

M-mode and Doppler findings change significantly depending upon the position of the patient.

Differentiation from LA Thrombus

- A left atrial myxoma needs to be differentiated from a thrombus at this site. Unlike a myxoma, a LA thrombus is close to the LA posterior wall, not pedunculated and it stays in the atrial cavity. It is rounded in shape with a more echogenic centre (old thrombus) and the mitral valve is often diseased.
- The differences between a left atrial thrombus and myxoma are enumerated in Table 15.1.

Table 15.1: Differences between LA thrombus and LA myxoma		
	LA thrombus	*LA myxoma*
Site	Posterior wall	Atrial septum
Attachment	Free	Pedunculated
Shape	Rounded	Lobulated
Echogenicity	Echogenic centre	Echolucent centre
Prolapse in MV	Rare	Often
Mitral valve	Diseased	Normal

Differentiation from Other Conditions

- On the basis of 2-D echo, myxoma needs to be differentiated from a left atrial thrombus (see above). On M-mode and Doppler echo, myxoma resembles mitral stenosis from which it can be differentiated by subtle features (see above). When the myxoma prolapses into mitral valve inflow, it can produce the auscultatory findings of mitral stenosis.

- The constitutional features of myxoma such as fever, arthralgia and anaemia need to be differentiated from those due to other clinical conditions such as bacterial endocarditis, collagen disorders and occult malignancy.

CARDIAC THROMBI

Types of Cardiac Thrombi

Atrial Thrombus

A. Left
B. Right

Ventricular Thrombus

A. Cavity
B. Mural

Left Atrial Thrombus

Requisites:	— diseased mitral valve
	— large left atrium
	— atrial arrhythmia
Predisposing conditions:	— mitral stenosis
	— prosthetic valve
	— atrial fibrillation
Locations:	— posterior atrial wall
	— free-floating (ball-valve)
	— left atrial appendage.
Other LA masses:	— left atrial myxoma
	— dilated coronary sinus

	—	flail mitral leaflet.
	—	reverberation artefact (calcific mitral annulus)
Linear LA structures:	—	cortriatriatum
	—	supravalvular ring
	—	anomalous pulm. veins.

Right Atrial Thrombus

Requisites:	—	indwelling venous line
	—	spread along vena cava (IVC)
Predisposing conditions:	—	Swan-Ganz catheter
	—	renal-cell carcinoma
Appearance:	—	pop-corn on string
Other RA masses:	—	right atrial myxoma
	—	metastatic tumour
	—	Chiari network (congenital remnant)
	—	Eustachian valve (guarding IVC orifice)
Linear RA structures:	—	Swan-Ganz catheter
	—	right pacing lead.

Echo Features of an Atrial Thrombus

- On 2-D imaging, an atrial thrombus appears as an echo-bright rounded mass arising from the posterior atrial wall or floating freely (Fig. 15.3). A thrombus in the left atrial appendage is more readily identified on transoesophageal echocardiography (TOE).
- A left atrial thrombus needs to be differentiated from a myxoma at this site by the features mentioned in Table (see above). A thrombus is rounded, freely

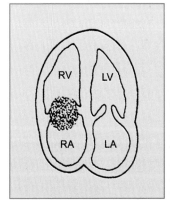

Fig. 15.3: Apical 4-chamber view showing a mass in the right atrium prolapsing through the tricuspid valve. This patient had a renal carcinoma that had spread along the inferior vena cava

mobile with an echogenic centre while a myxoma is lobulated, pedunculated with an echolucent centre.

- A rotatory motion of blood in the left atrium occurs when blood from pulmonary veins meets stagnant atrial blood. It produces a swirling 'smoke-like' pattern of echodensities within the left atrium due to clumping of RBCs (rouleaux formation) which become more echo-reflective. This is known as the 'whirlpool sign' or "spontaneous contrast effect". These signs indicate the presence of or a propensity towards genuine thrombus formation.

- A ball-valve thrombus can rarely obstruct the mitral valve orifice and prove fatal. When identified, it is an indication for urgent surgical intervention (Fig. 15.4).

- In a patient of mitral stenosis with atrial fibrillation who presents with a stroke due to cerebral embolism, it can be safely presumed that there is a left atrial thrombus. Failure to demonstrate an atrial thrombus could be due to its small size, location in the atrial

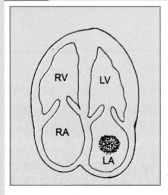

Fig. 15.4: Apical 4-chamber view showing a free-floating ball-valve thrombus in the left atrial cavity

appendage or due to the fact that it has already embolized.

VENTRICULAR THROMBUS

Requisites:	— dilated ventricular cavity
	— reduced wall contractility
	— stagnation of blood flow.
Predisposing conditions:	— dilated cardiomyopathy
	— myocardial infarction
	— ventricular aneurysm
Types:	— pedunculated (ball-like)
	— laminated (mural)
Other LV masses:	— LV tumour
	— papillary muscle
	— technical artefact
	— LV false tendon
Other RV masses:	— RV tumour
	— technical artefact
	— RV moderator band.

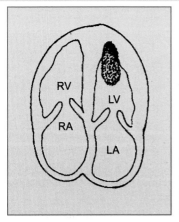

Fig. 15.5: Apical 4-chamber view showing a pedunculated thrombus protruding into the left ventricular cavity

Echo Features of Ventricular Thrombus

- On 2-D imaging, a pedunculated ventricular thrombus appears as a rounded mobile mass with a stalk, which protrudes into the ventricular cavity (Fig. 15.5). The mobility of the thrombus is not synchronous with the ventricular wall. The thrombus may be highly echogenic due to calcification or variable in echodensity due to necrotic areas. In the latter case, it is more likely to embolize.

- A mural ventricular thrombus is a flat, laminated mass, contiguous with the ventricular wall with which it moves synchronously (Fig. 15.6). It is more echogenic than the adjacent myocardium and less likely to embolize than a mobile thrombus. A fresh thrombus of recent origin may be isoechoic with the adjacent myocardium.

- Sometimes, waves of cloudy echoes drift in a swirling pattern representing stagnant blood and creating

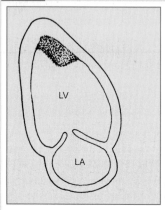

Fig. 15.6: Apical 2-chamber view showing a laminated thrombus contiguous with the ventricular wall

boundaries of acoustic impedance and increased echogenicity. They represent a heightened tendency towards genuine thrombus formation.

Differentiation from Other Ventricular Masses

- Mural thrombus can be distinguished from localized myocardial thickening since myocardium thickens during systole while a thrombus does not.
- Thrombus can be differentiated from a tumour by the fact that adjacent wall motion is almost always abnormal in case of a thrombus and often normal in case of tumour.
- Thrombus always has a clear identifiable edge while an artefact caused by stagnant blood does not. On colour Doppler, the flow profile stops abruptly at the edge of a thrombus but not at the edge of an artefact.

CHAPTER SIXTEEN

THROMBOEMBOLIC DISEASES

A fairly common question asked, when an echo is requested in a patient with transient ischemic attack or cerebral stroke is: Is there a cardiac source of embolism?

Indications for Echo in TIA/Stroke

1. To make or confirm a diagnosis associated with risk of thromboembolism such as:
   a. mitral stenosis, left atrial dilatation and atrial fibrillation
   b. prosthetic mitral/aortic valve, mitral valve prolapse
   c. dilated left ventricle, hypokinesia and ventricular aneurysm (see Intracardiac Masses).
2. To detect a direct source of embolism from the heart such as:
   a. left atrial thrombus
   b. left atrial myxoma
   c. mitral/aortic vegetation (see Intracardiac Masses and Endocardial Diseases).
3. To detect an indirect source of peripheral emboli such as:
   a. patent foramen ovale with atrial septal aneurysm allowing passage of venous thrombus from right to left (see Congenital Heart Diseases)
   b) aortic atheroma in the descending thoracic aorta that is large, mobile, pendunculated and ulcerated on its surface (see Aortic Diseases).

Who Should Have an Echo?

Not every patient who has had a TIA or Stroke needs an echo. However, it is certainly important in the following situations:

- Abrupt occlusion of a major peripheral or visceral artery.
- Young patient (< 50 years) with cerebral infarction
- Older patient (> 50 years) without evidence of cerebrovascular disease or any other obvious cause of CVA
- Strong clinical suspicion of cardiac embolism e.g. recurrent peripheral or cerebral embolic events.
- Clinical evidence of relevant structural heart disease e.g. mitral stenosis, or dilated left ventricle.
- Clinical suggestion of cardiac conditions causing embolism e.g. endocarditis or left atrial myxoma.
- Abnormal ECG findings indicating underlying heart disease e.g. Q waves, loss of R waves, ST-T changes or arrhythmias like atrial fibrillation and ventricular tachycardia.

Who Should Have a Transoesophageal Echo?

Many a time, a cardiac source of embolism is evident on conventional transthoracic echo. A subsequent transoesophageal echo is indicated in the following situations:

- Young patient (< 50 years) with TIA / stroke even in the absence of clinical cardiac abnormalities.
- Older patient (> 50 years) with no other cause of TIA/stroke.
- A normal or inconclusive transthoracic scan with strong clinical suspicion of cardiac embolism
  The following rare conditions can only be diagnosed by a transoesophageal echo:
- Occult left atrial myxoma

- Left atrial appendage thrombus
- Left atrial spontaneous contrast effect
- Patent foramen ovale with atrial septal aneurysm
- Aortic atheroma in the descending thoracic aorta.

Who Should NOT Have an Echo?

An echo is not indicated in TIA or stroke in the following situations:

- When there is evidence of intrinsic cerebrovascular disease sufficient to cause the clinical event e.g. more than 70% carotid stenosis on Doppler scan
- When the results of echocardiography will not influence therapeutic decisions e.g. diagnosing patent foramen ovale in a patient already on anticoagulants.

Thromboembolism in Mitral Stenosis

- The risk of thromboembolism in mitral stenosis is very high, particularly if atrial fibrillation is present and more so if it is intermittent. Mitral stenosis can be safely assumed to be the cause of cerebral infarction even in the absence of a demonstrable left atrial thrombus (too small for detection, atrial appendage thrombus, already embolized thrombus).
- In such patients anticoagulation can be initiated right-away provided there is no systemic contraindication to anticoagulants and cerebral haemorrhage has been excluded by a cranial CT scan.
- Occasionally, an echo may show a large left atrial ball thrombus which is an indication for urgent surgery.

CHAPTER SEVENTEEN

SYSTEMIC DISEASES

The Echo abnormalities observed in certain systemic diseases are enumerated in this section. It must be remembered that only some (not all) of the echo features may be present in a given case.

Diabetes Mellitus

- Effects of coexistent hypertensive heart disease.
- Effects of coexistent coronary artery disease.
- Left ventricular diastolic dysfunction (early stage)
- Left ventricular systolic dysfunction (late stage)
- Diabetic cardiomyopathy—systolic or diastolic

Hypothyroidism

- Left ventricular hypertrophy (eccentric)
- Left ventricular systolic dysfunction
- Pericardial effusion (minimal)

Chronic Anaemia

- Left ventricular hypertrophy (eccentric)
- Left ventricular dilatation (volume overload)
- Left ventricular diastolic dysfunction.

Chronic Renal Failure

- Pericardial effusion (uraemic)
- Left ventricular systolic dysfunction.
- Effects of coexistent hypertensive disease.
- Effects of coexistent coronary disease.

Malignant Disorder

- Pericardial effusion (metastatic or haematogenous)

- Cardiac tumour (direct invasion or metastasis)
- Non-infective (merantic) endocarditis

Collagen Disorder

- Pericarditis and effusion
- Myocardial infiltration
- Valvular regurgitation
- Non-infective (Libman-Sacks) endocarditis.

HIV Infection

- Dilated cardiomyopathy and myocarditis
- Pericardial effusion and tamponade
- Infective endocarditis (bacterial or fungal)
- Non-infective (merantic) endocarditis.
- Cardiac metastases from Kaposi's sarcoma
- Pulmonary hypertension and right ventricular dysfunction (recurrent chest infection).

INDEX

READER SUGGESTIONS SHEET

Please help us to improve the quality of our publications by completing and returning this sheet to us.

Title/Author: **ECHO MADE EASY** *by* **Dr Atul Luthra**

Your name and address:

Phone and Fax:

e-mail address:

How did you hear about this book? [please tick appropriate box (es)]

☐ Direct mail from publisher   ☐ Conference

☐ Bookshop   ☐ Book review

☐ Lecturer recommendation   ☐ Friends

☐ Other (please specify)   ☐ Website

Type of purchase: ☐ Direct purchase   ☐ Bookshop   ☐ Friends

Do you have any brief comments on the book?

Please return this sheet to the name and address givenbelow.

JAYPEE BROTHERS
MEDICAL PUBLISHERS (P) LTD
EMCA House, 23/23B Ansari Road, Daryaganj
New Delhi 110 002, India